THE SPECTRUM OF HOPE

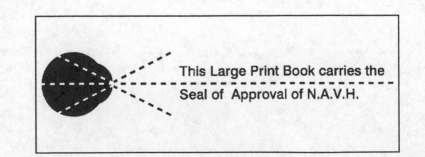

This Large Print Book carries the
Seal of Approval of N.A.V.H.

THE SPECTRUM OF HOPE

AN OPTIMISTIC AND NEW APPROACH TO ALZHEIMER'S DISEASE AND OTHER DEMENTIAS

GAYATRI DEVI, MD

THORNDIKE PRESS
A part of Gale, a Cengage Company

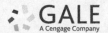

GALE
A Cengage Company

Farmington Hills, Mich • San Francisco • New York • Waterville, Maine
Meriden, Conn • Mason, Ohio • Chicago

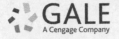

LIBRARY OF CONGRESS CIP DATA ON FILE.
CATALOGUING IN PUBLICATION FOR THIS BOOK
IS AVAILABLE FROM THE LIBRARY OF CONGRESS

ISBN-13: 978-1-4328-4647-3 (hardcover)
ISBN-10: 1-4328-4647-7 (hardcover)

Published in 2018 by arrangement with Algonquin Books of Chapel
Hill, a division of Workman Publishing Co., Inc.

Printed in Mexico
2 3 4 5 6 7 22 21 20 19 18

For my incredible daughter, Ginny.
May she find the practice of medicine
as wondrous as I have.

ACKNOWLEDGMENTS

Thanks to my agent, Laura Yorke, for many things — her fine wit, her quick intelligence, her love of "Old Cubans," her astounding loyalty, her indefatigable and super editing skills, and her belief in me.

Thanks to my dear friend Harry Lodge, who was involved in editing the nascent version, for being a fantastic colleague and internist, for his endearingly refractory nerdiness, and for sending me many of the patients whom you will meet.

Thanks to Rae Alexandra, for patiently transcribing my dictations, for reading aloud the final product in her glorious Welsh accent so I could hear how the stories sounded, for her keen sense of irony, her wonderful editing suggestions, and her fierce love of Besito and all things canine.

Thanks to Workman Publishing and Suzie

7

Bolotin for embracing and supporting the idea of this book from the get-go, and to Margot Herrera for being a sounding board and editor, and for asking the right, detail-oriented questions.

Finally, I would like to thank my patients — my adored, wonderful patients — and their caregivers. They continue to teach me so much — humbling me with their courage, strengthening me with their resilience, and inspiring me with their boundless generosity of spirit. To them, I owe my unbridled joy in the art and practice of medicine, and to them, in truth, I owe this book.

CONTENTS

INTRODUCTION:
A NEW PERSPECTIVE ON
ALZHEIMER'S DISEASE

"I feel like I am being completely controlled," said my 78-year-old patient Mary, a retired college professor with a brunette bob that neatly framed her dark eyes. She looked sadly at me, adding, "What I say makes no difference. Every aspect of my life is being managed. What is the point of living if things are going to go on like this?"

Her mood that day was very different from when I'd last seen her. What had happened in the interim? I soon found out. Her ophthalmologist, at the behest of Mary's daughters, had told her to stop driving.

"Her vision isn't good anymore," said one of Mary's daughters, who had accompanied her mother to my office. "And Dr. Smith felt that Mom wasn't safe behind the wheel."

"But my eyesight hasn't changed in ten years," Mary shot back. "I've had the same prescription since before your father died!"

Her daughter gave me that look that I have come to know so well, the *It's the dementia speaking; ignore what's being said* look. It's a look that I see daily on the faces of caregivers when patients assert that they are still working at the job they retired from years ago, when they insist they haven't had breakfast that morning, when they say that their children have stopped calling.

It's easy for me to recognize the *look,* and patients themselves quickly become aware of it as well. Not surprisingly, they are angry when their views, regardless of how erroneous they may be, are dismissed.

"Don't you give her that look!" Mary said, catching her daughter in the act. "You girls are treating me like I am a child. I am not a child, and I refuse to be treated like one!"

Mary turned back to me. "He acted like I was not in the room," she said, referring to her ophthalmologist. "He talked to my girls like I wasn't even there. His behavior was simply unacceptable. No one can keep me from driving. I want my car back. There is nothing that suddenly went so wrong with my vision that I can't drive."

In this case, it wasn't my patient's vision that prompted taking away the car keys — it was her dementia. Mary's daughters had asked the ophthalmologist to tell Mary her vision was impaired to keep her from driving.

Mary was the unwitting victim of the medical profession's difficulty understanding the variability characteristic of Alzheimer's disease. Having worked in the field of neurology and dementia for more than twenty years, I believe more and more that Alzheimer's is not a single disease entity, but rather a spectrum disorder that presents with different symptoms, progresses differently, and responds differently to treatment, with different prognoses, for each person. Mary's Alzheimer's was different from the Alzheimer's that affected Jack or Jill or Mike, just as Susan's stroke was different from Sam's. Post-stroke, Susan may be able to drive but unable to speak, whereas Sam may be able to give a toast at the Friars Club but needs crutches to get up to do so. Alzheimer's too affects different parts of the brain in different people, despite the fact that almost everyone with the disease eventually develops significant memory problems. So Mary's driving skills may have been unaffected by her Alzheimer's even though she may have trouble finding words. And Jack may have had some fender benders as the result of his Alzheimer's, despite remaining the life of the party. Jill's Alzheimer's may progress rapidly and aggressively, while Mike's might progress slowly.

Unfortunately, the differences between the various subcategories of Alzheimer's are lost when patients get tossed into the general diagnostic inbox. Although some patients with Alzheimer's become completely immobilized, most patients on the spectrum are living in the community, babysitting a grandchild, finishing up chores, or possibly even running for president of the United States (as we will read later). However, because Alzheimer's is still a poorly understood disease and because one's recall bias tends toward severe cases, the people we remember with the condition are often mute and using a wheelchair, suffering from advanced illness. When we think about the condition, we will not recall the absent-minded storekeeper or the lawyer who did a good job with cross-examining the witness on the stand. We have not yet learned to associate Alzheimer's disease with functioning individuals, although this is, in fact, the majority of patients.

Time and again, patients and caregivers who are worried about the potential ravages of Alzheimer's or another form of dementia make decisions based on fear or emotion, rather than on facts. I've come to realize that it is not only patients and family who react in this manner to a diagnosis of dementia — physicians and other health caregivers do too. I have been as guilty of this as anyone else. Patients themselves, confused and unsure about what to expect, may decide to fold up their lives like used notebooks and file themselves away. In allowing this to happen, we are doing ourselves and society a disservice, depriving patients with dementia and their communities of years of fulfillment, pleasure, and purpose-driven lives.

As I mentioned, I view Alzheimer's as a spectrum disorder. Furthermore, Alzheimer's is a *multifactorial* disease, which means that there can be many reasons that someone develops symptoms. In some cases, genetics may play a role, but lifestyle choices and myriad other factors can also lead to the condition. That one of a set of identical twins can get Alzheimer's while the other stays healthy is testament to this fact.

Because so many factors can contribute to a person developing symptoms — and because Alzheimer's presents differently in each person — I believe in a treatment approach that is tailored to the person and the subtype of disease they have. One size does not fit all for diabetes or strokes, which are other multifactorial illnesses, and one size does not fit all for Alzheimer's.

In the sixteen chapters that follow, I address a variety of common issues that come up in the care of patients with Alzheimer's and other dementias and attempt to answer the many poignant questions that I have been asked over the years.

"Should I tell my family and friends about my diagnosis?" a grandfather of four asks.

"I love what I do! Can I keep working?" asks a surgeon.

"Can I stay in my apartment? Or do I have to move into a home?" wonders an 80-year-old woman without any family.

"Should my children take over my finances?" asks the meticulous accountant.

"Who says I can't drive?" asks Mary.

"If it's not safe for Mom to drive, how can I tell her in a way that doesn't break her spirit?" Mary's daughter asks.

"Alan has become paranoid," his wife tells me. "He thinks I am stealing his money. Why would I do that after forty years of marriage? It makes me so sad that he would think that! What should I do?"

"She screams when she gets into the shower, and it breaks my heart," a concerned husband says.

"He doesn't think he has any problems

with his memory. He won't go to the doctor!" a son says in frustration.

"Sally keeps asking to go home, even though we are at home," Ed says.

The questions and concerns are endless. I try to be prepared with answers wrought from science and experience.

The fundamental question is this: *How can a person maintain dignity even as aspects of who they are begin to fragment and dissolve?* In pursuit of an answer, I have filled the pages that follow with practical advice on how to tailor one's approach to Alzheimer's and other types of dementia to suit the patient and their particular Alzheimer's experience. My goal is not to paint a rosy picture of Alzheimer's but a realistic one based on my practice.

MY APPROACH

I approach the subject of Alzheimer's personally, highlighting dilemmas I've encountered with real-life patients, caregivers, and situations over the course of my two-plus decades in practice. I also draw upon my experience serving as a consultant to New York State's Committee on Physician Health, where I assess the competence of our licensed physicians with cognitive issues and dementia. The information in this book will be helpful to both patients and their caregivers.

To protect my patients' and their caregivers' privacy, I have changed all identifying information. I am a rather formal person in my practice, preferring to address patients as Mr., Ms., Doctor, or Professor, but for the purposes of the book, I've given most patients first names for ease of reading.

Dementia is an umbrella term addressing all types of progressive cognitive loss, whereas *Alzheimer's* is a particular type of dementia and the most common. However, throughout the book, I use the terms *Alzheimer's* and *dementia* interchangeably.

The first several chapters deal with these questions: Do I have Alzheimer's disease? If yes, then what? How do I treat it? Whom should I tell? Can I keep working? Can I keep living in my home? Are there any specific challenges that women with memory loss face? Will I pass this on to my children and grandchildren?

The second set of chapters deals with some of the common symptoms that accompany Alzheimer's and how best to address them, as patients and as caregivers. Such symptoms can include depression, anxiety, apraxia, paranoia, personality changes, and wandering behavior. Then

20

there are a couple of chapters that focus on the challenges that caregivers face, including loneliness, depression, and often, a profound sense of guilt.

Next are chapters on end of life, which frankly apply to all of us and not just those of us with Alzheimer's. Here we look at whether medical illnesses are better treated at the hospital or at home as we age, how to deal with our idiosyncrasies as we get older, and how to die at home, which is what most of us prefer. Finally, I end with my own reflections as a physician taking care of patients with dementia, exploring how a field that many consider depressing has given me joy, solace, and fulfillment over all these years.

My purpose here is not to produce a comprehensive and exhaustive tome that covers every aspect of Alzheimer's, but rather a profoundly personal volume that deals with the most common daily problems that patients and their families encounter in their journey through life with dementia. I aim to address these problems from a patient-centered perspective that may not be as readily available in other comprehensive texts, and in doing so, I hope to be able to change the way people view the disease.

Finally, I would like to apologize in advance should I offend anyone's sensibilities, whether caregiver or patient, with my points of view. The opinions here are mine alone. As one of my wonderfully wise mentors, Dr. Roger Cracco, who was then chairman of the department of neurology, told me in the first month of my medical internship twenty-nine years ago, "Gayatri, fifty percent of what you are taught in medicine is wrong and fifty percent is right. The problem is, none of us know which is which. Only time will tell." This was humbling, coming from someone so accomplished and learned, and it is a lesson I keep close to my heart. So forgive me my transgressions, which are based on what I currently believe to be true.

CHAPTER 1
DO I HAVE ALZHEIMER'S?
IDENTIFYING MEMORY DISORDERS AND THE IMPORTANCE OF EARLY DIAGNOSIS

"If I find out I have Alzheimer's, I will commit suicide," exclaimed a woman I met at a cocktail party when she discovered what I did for a living. "I don't want to be a burden to my family." She was in her seventies and explained that she had recently noticed that her memory was slipping and she was having trouble finding words.

"First, we don't know if Alzheimer's is the cause of your problems," I said, offering a little impromptu advice. "And second, even if you have Alzheimer's, there are many things that can be done to keep it from progressing."

"I find that hard to believe!" the woman told me flatly. "That's not what I have heard and read."

Unfortunately, this rather common view prevents people with memory loss from

23

seeking help. Memory loss can arise from a number of conditions, including normal aging, hormone imbalance, side effects from medication, and strokes, as well as from dementias such as Alzheimer's. However, because of the fear of discovering that their memory loss might be caused by Alzheimer's, many people avoid or postpone getting evaluated. Such delays prevent treatment of easily addressed conditions and allow illnesses like Alzheimer's to affect more areas of the brain, at which point it becomes harder to stabilize. Most don't realize that, as with any other chronic illness, the earlier a diagnosis of Alzheimer's is made and treatment is started, the better the long-term prognosis.

In fact, studies of patients seen in internists' offices typically find that between 90 and 97 percent of those with mild dementia and 50 percent of those with moderate dementia remain undiagnosed by their physicians. A number of factors may be responsible for this low level of diagnosis. Some patients may not think enough of the memory loss to complain about it or may attribute it to factors such as stress or medication. Others may fear telling their physician about memory complaints and getting a dreaded diagnosis of dementia. Yet others may fear the loss of their job, familial upheaval, or even, as I have discovered, the loss of the respect of their longtime physician. I have had patients who have refused to let their internists know about their dementia diagnosis for years, concealing even their memory medications, because "I don't want to be treated differently." Finally, this tremendous level of underdiagnosis may be caused by some physicians not being as responsive to memory complaints or signs in their patients as they might be to more straightforward problems such as chest pain or constipation.

This not only does the patients a disservice by not getting them treatment for curable causes of memory loss, but it also prevents those with Alzheimer's from getting the early treatment that can make a real difference. Further complicating things, like my cocktail party acquaintance, most people believe that even if they do have Alzheimer's, there are no effective treatments for the condition. Additionally, most folks do not realize that *Alzheimer's is a spectrum disorder, not a single disease.* Alzheimer's disease presents and progresses differently in different people, meaning that a diagnosis of Alzheimer's is not necessarily the disaster that many of us imagine it to be. At some point, ideally in the near future, scientists will be able to parse out different subtypes of the condition that make up the Alzheimer's spectrum, thus helping to allay the fear of this diagnosis.

Already, there are subtypes of Alzheimer's defined by biological markers, genetics, and clinical symptoms. These subtypes progress differently, behaving almost like different illnesses despite the common pathology. Patients with Alzheimer's beginning at a young age, say in their forties and fifties, have a specific set of associated genetic mutations, develop a different pattern of symptoms, and progress rapidly to death. On the other end of the Alzheimer's spectrum are older men and women with brains that are pathologically identical to Alzheimer's brains but without any symptoms of the condition. Can we then say that this is all the same disease? It seems more plausible that Alzheimer's is a constellation of different types of disease that contribute to a final common pathology with markedly different presentations, treatment responses, and outcomes.

Contrary to popular belief, most people with Alzheimer's disease are not going to forget who they are or the names of those they love. Most men and women with Alzheimer's disease will live at home and die at home. Because the brain is a complex organ, even patients with the same subtype of Alzheimer's can present with different symptoms. Depending on the area of the brain that is first affected by the dementia pathology, some patients may notice difficulty with arithmetic, whereas others may have trouble reading; some people may have trouble finding words, and others may have difficulty driving. The early symptoms of dementia are as varied as the brain's many functions.

As one of my friends who works in the field put it, "Twenty million people with Alzheimer's have twenty million types of Alzheimer's," alluding to the individual variability of the disease. Unlike organs such as the heart, which pumps blood, or the bladder, which holds urine, the brain is responsible for a multitude of functions, overseeing not only the work of the bladder and the heart, but also how to kiss, dance, and drive a car. Bladder disease affects one function, whereas brain disease can affect hundreds of different abilities.

Because of the brain's versatility as an organ, I find it hard to answer questions about the severity or stages of Alzheimer's disease, particularly early in the disease's course.

"What stage am I in?" a patient might ask.

"I can't give you an overall stage," I might answer. "Your memory is poor, but your language skills are excellent, as are your life skills." In contrast, diseases of organs such as the lung or the liver are easier to stage, because of the organs' singular functions.

JOE'S ALZHEIMER'S

Joe, a patrician-looking, city-born-and-bred 73-year-old, came to see me with his stylish wife and their grown-up daughter. He was a money manager in charge of more than a billion dollars in assets. Recently Joe's memory had been fading, and trades and transactions — which used to come as naturally to him as breathing — had started causing him trouble. No one had commented about his difficulties on the job, but because he owned his firm, he was concerned that people were hesitant about correcting the boss.

"I was born with an extremely good brain and I've utilized it very well," Joe said. "But in the last couple of years or so, I've been forgetting. I watch a movie and lose the thread of it. I drive right past my destination. I used to have a fantastic vocabulary, and now I search for words. I think my brain cells are dying."

Attesting to his eloquence, Joe summed up by saying, "I see a consistent failure in cognition."

"Joe is the smartest man I've ever met," his wife added. "He makes numbers dance! He used to have an incredible memory, but it has become unreliable. The other day, he couldn't remember our home alarm system's security code, a number he's punched in a thousand times." She paused. "That's not Joe. Joe can recite telephone numbers from memory. He's never needed to write down a single phone number. Now he's forced to write everything down, and he relies on his secretary to help him."

The couple's daughter was very concerned as well. She noticed that her father, a man who had effortlessly led a large, successful, and highly regarded financial firm for forty years, had become increasingly forgetful. The three of them were at my office because Joe's astute internist had expressed concern that Joe might be developing Alzheimer's disease or another type of dementia.

It turned out that the internist was right — Joe did have Alzheimer's. I discovered this after I performed a thorough evaluation and a laboratory workup, including a magnetic resonance imaging scan, or MRI.

Fortunately, Joe had several things going for him that were associated with a better prognosis. He was still working, meaning that he was keeping his brain active. He appeared to be handling the demands of his job, which meant that the pathology was not yet significantly affecting his functioning. He had a supportive family and social network that kept him from social isolation. All these factors meant he had a good *cognitive* reserve, which kept his brain resilient. He also had good *brain* reserve because he was physically in good shape. He exercised twice a week, which kept his heart healthy and increased blood flow through his brain, making for a more robust brain. In the next chapter we will learn more about how these two types of reserve — cognitive and brain — function as mental "money in the bank" and help stave off the effects of Alzheimer brain pathology.

Finally, Joe was motivated to seek any and all available treatments, both those already approved for Alzheimer's and those that were still "off-label" but seemed promising. Off-label interventions have been approved by the Food and Drug Administration (FDA) for use in one or more illnesses, but not for the condition being treated. For example, although many chemotherapy drugs are FDA-approved to treat one type of cancer, they are commonly and legally used "off-label" to treat other types of cancer. After hearing his diagnosis, he said, "Throw the book at me! What do I have to lose? Let's do everything we can, and if we fail? Well, at least we tried."

So we started Joe on a combination of medication and a brain stimulation regimen designed to bolster his cognitive and brain reserves and keep his brain resilient even as the pathological deposits in his brain increased.

That was seven years ago. Joe is 80 now. How is he doing? Well, recently, I got a call from a new cardiologist whom Joe had seen at his internist's behest, for a problem unrelated to his memory. The cardiologist was outraged.

"What do you mean Joe has Alzheimer's?" he asked me disbelievingly. "His memory is better than mine! There's nothing wrong with him. I think you should redo all the tests you've been doing, because I do not believe this man has Alzheimer's."

What Joe's cardiologist did not realize was that Joe had already undergone numerous tests that all pointed to the same diagnosis. He had even had spinal fluid analysis, which was positive for the abnormal brain deposits that are seen in Alzheimer's disease. Joe had been serially tested for the previous seven years and had shown remarkable stability in most areas, such as visuospatial skills, and even improvement in others, such as language, although his memory remained poor. Some may consider it heresy to speak of improvement in Alzheimer's, but Joe unequivocally showed a positive response to his treatment.

Interestingly, Joe had more insight into his cardiologist's irate reaction to the diagnosis than I did. When I recounted the conversation to Joe, he said, "My cardiologist's wife died of Alzheimer's. I understand she was quite ill and spent the last year in a nursing home. He is old-school, and I don't think he understands or believes that some people with Alzheimer's can keep functioning with the right treatment."

Despite the pervasive belief that Alzheimer's is a one-way street to inexorable decline, Joe's situation will be familiar to any physician who has spent several years dealing with patients who have the condition. Some patients do, in fact, *improve* with treatment, and many patients do stay stable. When one recognizes Alzheimer's as a spectrum disorder rather than as a single disease entity, this becomes more under-standable. The wonderful thing was that Joe continued to work and find utility in his life. He eventually relinquished managing his firm, but he stayed on in a part-time capac-ity. By the time he turned 80, he was spend-ing more time in Florida, and it felt natural at this stage in his life to be cutting down on work. Joe is proof that living a highly functional life despite having Alzheimer's disease is possible, and he continues to do so as this book goes to print.

What stage of dementia is Joe in? As I mentioned earlier, I personally dislike stag-ing, because I find it to be of limited utility in terms of prognosis or thinking about the disease in an individual person. Instead, here's how I would describe where Joe falls on the Alzheimer's spectrum: He has slowly progressive Alzheimer's with excellent language skills, moderate memory loss, and good life skills (which comprise tasks impor-tant for independent living, like driving and shopping). Joe had a good overall prognosis because of his high levels of cognitive and brain reserve and positive response to treat-ment.

Tools for Making a Diagnosis of Alzheimer's

A good cognitive evaluation is composed of many parts. Here are some of the common components:

- A thorough physical examination for treatable causes of memory loss, like thyroid disease
- A neurologic and psychiatric examination for conditions like stroke or depression, which may mimic dementia
- A review of the patient's medical history and medications, because certain medication side effects can mimic dementia
- A cognitive evaluation — testing for memory, language, and visuospatial skills — to get a baseline "functional brain map," which helps with locating the patient on the Alzheimer's spectrum and guides prognosis and treatment
- A magnetic resonance imaging scan, or MRI, of the brain to look for tumors and evidence of silent strokes that may not be readily perceptible on examination
- Blood tests, including for Lyme disease and vitamin deficiencies, the symptoms of which can mimic dementia
- An electroencephalogram, or EEG, to see how the brain is functioning electrically, just like an electrocardiogram, or EKG,

34

looks at the heart's electrical activity. On rare occasions seizures can mimic dementia.

In some cases, depending on the clinical presentation, additional tests are done:
• Cerebrospinal fluid evaluation via a spinal tap to evaluate for unusual brain infections that can cause memory loss
• An Amyvid positron emission tomography (PET) functional imaging scan to evaluate the extent of amyloid plaque deposit in the brain, which is associated with Alzheimer's
• A fluorodeoxyglucose PET functional imaging scan to evaluate glucose use in the brain, which is reduced in those parts of the brain that are affected by disease

MEGAN'S ALZHEIMER'S

Not many people are aware of outcomes as positive as Joe's. For the most part, the Alzheimer's stories that crowd the general consciousness are hopeless worst-case scenarios. Another of my patients, 69-year-old Megan, voiced the common negative misconception.

"What will happen to me?" she asked me tearfully. "Do I need to put my affairs in order? I don't want to live if I lose my mind.

I think I will fly off to one of those countries where I can kill myself legally before I allow that to happen." It was a few weeks after I had first seen her for her memory complaints. She had undergone an extensive evaluation, and I had given her a diagnosis of slowly progressive Alzheimer's disease with mild memory loss and excellent language and life skills, with a likely good prognosis, given her high levels of brain and cognitive reserve.

Megan lived alone and had no children or family, other than distant cousins who lived on the opposite coast. She prided herself on her smarts and relied on them. Although she had only an eighth-grade education, she had worked her way up to become the chief administrator for an extremely prestigious private firm. In her position, there was little room for error. If Megan made a mistake, it was observable not only to her boss, but to all of her junior staff. By the very nature of her job, Megan's performance was being constantly and inadvertently assessed by many people.

Megan first noticed her brain wasn't as sharp as it had been when she began having mild difficulty remembering things, including appointments. As someone who had had prodigious organizational abilities, this development was alarming to her. The change had been apparent to no one but herself, but she came in for an evaluation to find out what was happening, as a precaution. This pragmatism exemplified Megan's matter-of-fact approach to life, so different from many others, who, when experiencing cognitive changes, might be tempted to "bury their head in the sand." Once I realized Megan had abnormalities on her neurocognitive evaluation, we performed a scan that indeed confirmed the presence of the plaques associated with Alzheimer's disease. Megan's vigilant, no-nonsense approach paid off, and the disease was diagnosed very early in its course, which is important for effective treatment.

Megan expressed her panicked thoughts about assisted suicide just as she was about to start her new treatment regimen.

"How am I going to do?" she asked.

"I don't know exactly how you are going to do at this point," I replied. "You may be someone who stabilizes with treatment. You might be able to keep working into your late seventies. Perhaps even into your eighties. But you might also be someone who doesn't respond to treatment. I won't know for sure until we reevaluate you after at least six months, but I think you will do well because of your excellent health, because you have an active and engaged brain to start with, and because we are beginning treatment early. You were proactive and brave enough to seek an evaluation as quickly as you did, which gives us a greater chance of success. We are getting you started on treatment right away, and again, my sense is that you will do well." By treatment, I meant not just medication, but a whole set of behavioral and other interventions tailored to Megan's symptoms.

THE CURRENT VIEW OF TREATMENT OF ALZHEIMER'S DISEASE

Like many of my patients, Megan listened to me talk about positive outcomes with disbelief etched on her face. Although my patients want to believe that treatment may help them, everything they've read and heard makes Alzheimer's seem like an inexorably progressive condition that decimates a person's mind and brain. The disease is presented as if it leaves each and every patient a physical shell of their former self, unable to recognize their loved ones, unable to appreciate life's simple pleasures, unable to remember anything, unable to do much of anything other than occupy space.

In fact, a diagnosis of Alzheimer's disease

does not often end that way, but few people are aware of this. This is because, as we read earlier, the overwhelming majority of patients with mild Alzheimer's and half of those with moderate disease go undiagnosed. Even when patients have received a diagnosis of Alzheimer's, the diagnosis is met with suspicion if they remain functional, as in Joe's case with his cardiologist. It's a damned if you do, damned if you don't, catch-22 situation. Only clearly impaired patients meet the public (and sometimes the physician's) idea of what Alzheimer's looks like. This is similar to saying that someone with cancer does not have cancer unless they are visibly ill, which we know to be untrue. This skewed mind-set about outcome also delays seeking help early, when treatment has the greatest effect.

An example that I like to give to demonstrate the futility of this type of thinking is diabetes, another multifactorial disease with multiple genetic causes affecting increasingly large portions of our population. There are people with diabetes who are unresponsive to multiple aggressive treatments, and there are people with diabetes whose symptoms can be controlled by dietary changes. But even though there are patients who can and do die from diabetes, no one assumes that every single person with that illness is going to end up a blind double amputee with strokes. Time and experience have allowed our understanding of diabetes to become both more accurate and more nuanced.

Take autism as another example. Not that long ago, few people thought of autism as a spectrum disorder. The public and physicians associated autistic patients with those at the severe end of the spectrum and did not appreciate the wide variations in the condition. Now, of course, we are aware that although some have significant impairment, more and more patients with functional autism (often called Asperger's syndrome) have been identified. We have grasped the heterogeneity of autism spectrum disorders. These changes in perception have been driven more by parents of children with autism educating the public than by the medical establishment. Such committed and fierce advocacy groups also exist for Alzheimer's. It is my hope that through education, the public perception of Alzheimer's can be changed as we work to remove the stigma associated with it, understand that it is a spectrum illness, and recognize that there are competent, high-functioning individuals with the condition.

BAD LUCK OR BAD GENES?

"What did I do? How did I get this?" patients often ask after receiving a diagnosis of Alzheimer's. "No one in my family has it."

Is getting Alzheimer's just bad luck, bad genes, bad environment, or something else? Depending on where one falls on the Alzheimer's spectrum, the answer varies. Let's use the diabetes analogy here again. There are people who have severe forms of diabetes who develop it as children — this type has a strong genetic component, requiring aggressive treatment, and patients sometimes die young, as a friend's son recently did at 28. However, the most common type of diabetes, reaching epidemic proportions in some countries, is a form associated with poor dietary choices, sedentary habits, and obesity, and usually appears later in life. A change in lifestyle can sometimes cure these cases. Similarly, genetics is a strong factor when Alzheimer's begins in younger ages, but many lifestyle factors contribute to the far more common Alzheimer's of older age. Being physically active and mentally and socially engaged helps delay the onset of symptoms. In fact, 60 percent of late-onset

41

Alzheimer's cases are thought to be preventable. Properly treating cardiovascular issues, including high blood pressure and heart disease, is another way to reduce risk. Even so, highly intellectual and physically active people can still develop the disease.

Some cases of Alzheimer's are inherited as aggressive familial illnesses, and on rare occasion they can occur in even very young adults, although we generally associate Alzheimer's with the elderly. The youngest patient with Alzheimer's I ever diagnosed, Theo, was only 29 when he developed symptoms, and he died in his thirties, unresponsive to treatment. You will meet Theo in a later chapter. Far more common are patients with Alzheimer's like Joe who develop it later in life and respond well to treatment. Some people with Alzheimer's refuse treatment after being diagnosed, and although a majority of them deteriorate in their cognitive abilities, some continue to function independently and die of other causes. In fact, there are people who have clear pathological evidence of Alzheimer's on brain autopsy but never develop clinical symptoms in their lives. What protected them? We think that a combination of good brain reserve, good cognitive reserve, and a unique immune system may help.

All of this helps explain why I had no definite answers yet for a distraught Megan directly after her diagnosis. I was able to tell her that there were indications that she might do well, because she was physically fit and had no cardiovascular risk factors or history of head injuries or strokes. This served to keep the estimated 80-plus billion nerve cells in Megan's brain — her brain reserve — healthy even as millions of her brain cells died weekly both from normal aging and from Alzheimer's. Although the idea of losing so many brain cells may be alarming, in fact, it is the connections between the cells more than the absolute number of cells that keep the brain functioning well. Symptoms from mild concussions, for example, arise more from disrupted connections than from cell death. And when certain brain areas are used less — say, those involved in cognitive tasks like reading or math — then connections in those areas become weaker, even if the number of brain cells remains unchanged. Conversely, practicing strengthens the connections between nerve cells, changing cobwebs into cables. Megan's hardwired neuronal cables and trillions of synaptic "switch" connections between her nerve cells — her cognitive reserve — would keep her brain functioning well, even as it was assaulted by Alzheimer's pathology.

Unfortunately, Megan's brain scan showed moderate to severe plaque deposits, which suggested that her brain pathology was far along. Also, her laboratory testing revealed a copy of the E4 variant of the APOE gene. This variant is associated with more rapid progression of the disease. At 69, Megan was relatively young, and she was in great physical health. This meant we needed to keep her brain functioning well for at least ten to fifteen years, based on her predicted life expectancy. After factoring in these variables, I thought that Megan would respond well to aggressive treatment, and she and I developed a plan, using both approved and off-label options. I let her know that we wouldn't be able to assess how she was responding and how her particular Alzheimer's was developing until she'd been treated for at least six months. Would I be right about Megan's response to treatment? We will find out in the next chapter.

When treating chronic conditions with varying clinical symptoms like Alzheimer's disease, it is crucial to wait an appropriate length of time before deciding whether to continue or discard a treatment. Patients can have days, weeks, and even months when they feel "sharp" and days, weeks, and months when they are "foggy." This may not be a reflection of worsening pathology but may be owing to another cause, such as depression, infection, or just the normal variation of our brain's abilities. We can all relate to having good days or weeks when we are on the ball and other days or weeks when we can't even recollect our friends' names, let alone what we had for breakfast. We can sometimes point to clear triggers like poor sleep as a culprit, but other times there is no rhyme or reason for such cognitive fluctuations. This is why I tell patients, most of whom are understandably anxious, that we have to wait some time to make sure that we are not interpreting the common fluctuations seen in the disease course as a particular response to treatment.

A SPECTRUM-BASED APPROACH TO ALZHEIMER'S

Over the past two-plus decades, I have seen several thousand patients with memory loss. I have had the honor and privilege of being able to follow many of them for years as they have improved, stayed stable, or declined. Nearly all of them had a complete evaluation when they first saw me, and many have had serial testing over the years. Based on this enormous amount of data, I have been able to come up with a method of categorizing patients on the spectrum that has been helpful to me and to my patients. My classification system allows me to view each person in terms of where they are on the Alzheimer's spectrum, and to determine prognosis and decide on appropriate treatment. I prefer at least two sets of data points over at least a six-month period to improve my prognostic accuracy, as I told Megan. Nevertheless, I am able to have a fairly good predictive idea of prognosis and response to treatment after a comprehensive baseline evaluation.

I factor in the patient's age, medical and family history, general health, brain reserve, cognitive reserve, laboratory and genetic testing, and current level of functioning. Younger age, a medical history with multiple cardiovascular risk factors, one or more affected family members, poor general fitness, genetic risk factors, laboratory markers of inflammation and other disease, and low brain and cognitive reserve are all associated with a poorer prognosis. (You will read about many of these risks for poorer prognosis as well as how to counteract them over the course of this book.) I also carefully review patients' performance on various neurocognitive tests, including language, memory, visuospatial ability, and what I call life or living skills. Such skills include the patient's ability to perform various activities of daily living, such as shopping, cooking, socializing, and getting around.

Based on all of this information, I make several decisions. First, I decide whether the person has rapidly progressive or slowly progressive Alzheimer's. In other words, I ask myself how quickly I estimate the disease will progress. Second, I evaluate the major cognitive areas — primarily language, memory, visuospatial, and social and life skills — in terms of the level to which each is affected or unaffected. This helps me better customize treatments to the patient and their subtype of Alzheimer's, rather than using a one-size-fits-all approach. Third, I determine with the patient what level of functioning they wish to maintain: Do they want to keep working, for example, or do they feel that they would like to switch tracks and retire, spending more time with family? Based on all these considerations, I formulate a treatment plan.

Although everyone is interested in maintaining as much cognitive functioning as possible, this needs to be weighed against the costs — in terms of time, finances, side effects, and sheer inconvenience — associated with more aggressive treatments for Alzheimer's. This risk-benefit analysis occurs with other chronic illnesses as well. For example, an athlete with an aggressive arthritic condition who wishes to continue competing will require far more rigorous intervention than one who is willing to give up the game.

"I CAN'T REMEMBER, SO I MUST BE STUPID."

The belief that "I must be stupid because I can't remember anything" is a common fallacy that occurs when we equate memory with intelligence. It can be prevented by a systematic approach to cognition in patients on the spectrum.

To distinguish and emphasize the difference between memory and general intellectual ability, I go over areas of functioning with patients and each area is rated as excellent, good, mild, moderate, or severe. This allows a patient and her family to understand, for example, that although she has severe memory loss, her life skill loss is mild and her language skills remain excellent.

I can then counter a patient's negative estimation of themselves in the face of their dementia. "How can you say you are stupid? It's true your memory is in the second percentile compared with other women in your age group, but your vocabulary is in the eightieth percentile. In a room of one thousand people your age without dementia, your vocabulary would be better than eight hundred of them!" Using a spectrum-based approach allows for both patients and caregivers to appreciate areas of strength and areas of weakness in a quantifiable way, and it helps them maintain confidence in their intellect despite a diagnosis of Alzheimer's.

A WIDER SPECTRUM

Although I have approached symptomatic Alzheimer's as a spectrum disorder for more than a decade, in 2012, the Alzheimer's Association and the National Institute of Aging corroborated my thinking, coming out with a new definition of Alzheimer's as a spectrum disorder. They based their definition on a combination of clinical signs and the presence of biological brain markers, focusing on plaque deposition. They defined preclinical Alzheimer's as a stage with the presence of plaque but no clinical symptoms, mild cognitive impairment as a stage with some objective symptoms and no functional issues, and Alzheimer's as the third stage. I subdivide this clinical third stage into my own two broad categories of rapidly and slowly progressive Alzheimer's. I further divide these two groups into subcategories defined by the type and degree to which functions are affected and the areas of the brain that are most involved.

This has proved to be a better system for me and my patients and their families, with more clinical utility and prognostic value, than thinking of the illness in broad stages of mild, moderate, or severe. I am confident that in the future, several subtypes of Alzheimer's disease will be better defined, allowing for tailored clinical trials and a deeper understanding of the spectrum as a whole. The teasing out of the subtypes within the Alzheimer's spectrum is already beginning among experts in the field. Patients with predominant visuospatial impairment, for example, may be diagnosed with posterior cortical atrophy, a subtype of Alzheimer's, whereas those with more language loss, many of whom show Alzheimer's pathology, may be diagnosed with primary progressive aphasia.

In this book, I will focus on the Alzheimer's part of the spectrum. I don't discuss mild cognitive impairment or preclinical Alzheimer's. These areas continue to be clarified and reclassified. Recent definition changes, for example, reclassified more than 93 percent of the cases formerly called "mild Alzheimer's" into the mild cognitive impairment category, highlighting the level to which the field is in flux. There is still much to learn about this group of illnesses, but this much is certain: Approaching Alzheimer's as a spectrum disorder allows for finer tuning of both diagnosis and treatment.

Here are two examples of the specific diagnoses I give patients based on the information I collect. Joe had slowly progressive Alzheimer's with moderate memory loss, excellent language skills, and good life skills, which in my experience is associated with a good prognosis and a good response to treatment. He wanted to maintain a high level of functioning, which warranted more aggressive treatment. Megan had slowly progressive Alzheimer's disease with mild memory loss and excellent language and life skills, with a likely good prognosis.

BELLA'S ALZHEIMER'S
Bella was 75 and managed my pension plan. She'd done an excellent job of it for more than a decade before she came in to see me one morning with her husband, concerned

that her memory was failing. Bella had a huge portfolio of pension funds for various large companies as well as for many individuals such as myself. She took pride in caring for them all very personally and once told me that she treated her clients' funds in exactly the same way that she would her own family's.

This attitude was one of the reasons that I had invested with Bella. I found her honest, intelligent, and hardworking. Now here she was at my office, not discussing my IRAs but worried that her mind was failing her. At first, I was taken aback because she was doing so well at her job, producing very successful returns. But Bella was insistent.

"My mother and her brother had memory problems," Bella said. "This has always been at the back of my mind. I look at something and I can't remember what it is — the TV remote, for example, or the carbon monoxide alarm. A couple of weeks ago I put in an order to sell when I should have bought. It was an easy mistake, but you have to check me out!"

We did. Unfortunately, Bella was right — she had been developing Alzheimer's disease. Much of what she had been worrying about now made sense to her. Bella had been having trouble remembering whom she was talking to on the phone. She would find herself stopping conversations midtrack. The words she intended to say would disappear as though she were the victim of a conjurer's trick, vanishing from within her throat even as she tried to speak them.

Bella had slowly progressive Alzheimer's with mild-moderate memory loss, mild language loss, and good life skills. She started taking medications approved for treating dementia and began a course of weekly physical and cognitive exercises. She also began to use off-label approved treatments, including magnetic brain stimulation, which is FDA-approved for depression and which, in my research, is beneficial in Alzheimer's. Within four to five months, she told me that she had regained a lot of her abilities and felt much better than she had in a long time. She still had some difficult days when she felt "foggy," but overall, she thought her symptoms had resolved. I confirmed Bella's observations after six months of treatment, by doing objective testing of her cognitive ability. Happily, she has stayed improved and, as of the writing of this book, Bella just celebrated her 80th birthday. She finally retired from the pension business a few months after these festivities, not because of cognitive issues but because she wanted to. As Bella put it, "It's about time I behave like the grandmother I am, and spend more time with my grandchildren."

CATHERINE'S ALZHEIMER'S

Although Joe and Bella have done very well, there are, of course, people who don't respond to treatment or who are not given the opportunity to receive adequate treatment.

One such patient was Catherine, a bubbly 53-year-old when she first came to see me. Slim and petite, with brown hair in a pixie cut, she lived with her husband and three teenage daughters. She told me that over the previous few years she had been having some difficulty finding words, and sometimes she forgot to walk Constance, her dog. She said that it was subtle enough that no one had really noticed, but Catherine realized something was happening to her. She had been working as a very successful fashion executive, living in a high-pressure world and thriving in it, but had stopped working three years before seeing me because she was concerned about her cognition.

Catherine had married her college sweetheart and raised her children in New York City. She simply couldn't think of living anywhere else in the world. Observing her effervescent personality in my office that hot summer afternoon, there wasn't a doubt in my mind that Catherine's symptoms were most consistent with menopause. I'd seen this often with women in their fifties. They would come to see me, terrified that they were developing Alzheimer's, and then we would find out that they actually had something curable, like menopause-related memory loss.

I was very much looking forward to having Catherine tested and then being able to reassure her that it wasn't what she thought. I wanted to be able to tell her that she was suffering from something far simpler, something temporary. Unfortunately, I wasn't able to do that.

Her initial tests included my usual workup: a laboratory and neurocognitive evaluation and an MRI, following the official criteria laid out by the National Institute of Neurological Diseases and Stroke. Although Catherine *was* menopausal, her performance on testing was suggestive of rapidly progressive Alzheimer's, with moderate memory impairment and mild language impairment. I was stunned. I did further confirmatory tests, including a PET scan, which showed evidence of reduced activity in the parts of the brain that are affected in Alzheimer's. I still couldn't believe it. Catherine presented as too functional. So I did a spinal tap, which came back positive for Alzheimer's, revealing evidence of significant buildup of the telltale plaques and tangles. (Tangles are the other pathological deposits seen in the brains of patients with Alzheimer's, and a scan for tangles will soon be commercially available.)

Although she'd known something was amiss, Catherine was dumbfounded — as was I. We both scrambled to get her treated as aggressively as possible: She was young, and as she said, "My girls haven't graduated high school, for heaven's sake!" Catherine had the kind of Alzheimer's, beginning before the age of 65, that is often, although not invariably, associated with a more aggressive course. She was all for trying any available treatments, including off-label ones that were not covered by her insurance, such as the ones that Joe, Bella, and Megan underwent.

However, her husband, Chad, was averse to any interventions that would involve the depletion of their finances. As a result, I tried to enroll Catherine in a variety of trials, which had the benefit of being free of charge and cutting-edge, because although there was a 50 percent chance that she would be on a placebo or "sugar-pill" treatment, there was a 50 percent chance that she would be on a potentially beneficial treatment. Chad was willing to go along with this, so I made some calls and had her evaluated.

Unfortunately for Catherine, her Alzheimer's was so atypical that the research center I had sent her to called and told me they were questioning her Alzheimer's diagnosis, despite the positive spinal tap tests, and suggested that perhaps she was suffering from depression. Because of this, they did not enroll her in the trials she was eligible for. Sadly, Catherine was too smart for her own good — she had done so well on the testing that no one at the center believed she actually had Alzheimer's disease. It was too early in the course of her illness for them to recognize it.

This also speaks to another difficulty in making a diagnosis of Alzheimer's disease: Some physicians make the diagnosis more readily than others. This may be confusing and alarming for the reader, but if there is ever any concern about the correctness of the diagnosis, a second opinion from another specialist should be obtained. Alternatively, if getting a second opinion is not feasible, retesting in a year to evaluate for progression consistent with Alzheimer's is another option. Retesting Catherine in a year would have confirmed her diagnosis to doubting Thomases, although unfortunately, she would have lost valuable treatment time. The earlier treatment is started, the better the ability to delay progression, even in those with a rapidly progressive course like Catherine's.

Seven years have passed, and now no one would doubt her diagnosis. The once vibrant Catherine doesn't speak much anymore, although she still gives me her brilliant smile every time she sees me. Her high brain and cognitive reserves, which served Bella and Joe so well, were no match for the virulence of her early-onset Alzheimer's.

Catherine's life has changed in other ways as well. Although she has remained married, Chad sold the family home and moved Catherine into her own apartment with a live-in aide while he moved into an apartment of his own. The initial idea had been to place Catherine in a nursing home, but I convinced Chad that having Catherine in her own place, with her dog, would be a better option. Chad began dating several years into Catherine's illness, although he was still very involved in her care. He accompanied her on doctor visits, was in charge of her medications, visited her several evenings a week, and kept close tabs on her emotional and physical state. Although her husband's dating may strike some people as callous, caregivers like Chad need to be understood, not vilified. Caregiving can be a tremendously lonely and draining task, and seeking companionship and solace is only human, as we will discuss at length later in the book (see Chapter 12). All three of Catherine's children graduated college and moved away to start lives of their own. These days, Catherine and her dog, Constance, live in an apartment with a lovely, vivacious caregiver, Elma, and the two of them are quite close. Catherine still makes funny comments sometimes, but when I ask her how many children she has, she can't really answer. When I ask her if she's married, sometimes she'll say yes, sometimes not. She still answers to her name. Parenthetically, Chad noted that the cost of his wife's care at home with an aide was less than the cost of placing her in a nursing home. I am glad, as this enables Catherine to stay in her familiar neighborhood and to continue activities she enjoys, like walking her dog. At-home care with paid attendants is not just the province of the wealthy. Medicaid, for example, will cover home care in New York State, from a few hours daily to round-the-clock. Such care may be more humane for the patient and less expensive for society at large than placement in a facility.

The sad thing is, Catherine is still physically very healthy, without any other chronic illness, making it inevitable that she will become a patient who simply devolves into the shell of Alzheimer's — the stereo-typical specter that many of us fear. Watching her rapid deterioration, it has become clear to me that she will soon be trapped in her body and long outlive her brain's ability to keep her functioning and engaged with the world. In all likelihood, Catherine will eventually die of pneumonia or another infection related to being bed-bound.

I do believe that had Catherine been able to avail herself of the treatments, off-label though they might have been, she may have maintained a higher quality of life for longer, even though she has a rapidly progressive, aggressive type of Alzheimer's. It should be noted that my only justification for that belief is a strong clinical sense and my professional experience. I have no proof of it.

Patients who progress to where Catherine did — not being able to tell me their children's names — constitute less than 5 percent of my practice. The vast majority of my patients are like Joe or Bella — functional and productive folks enjoying their families, friends, jobs, and lives. However, because people like Catherine are the ones in nursing homes — which is where Catherine would be had I not advocated for the alternative situation — this is the image that comes to mind when people think of Alzheimer's. They see only one aspect of the vast spectrum that is Alzheimer's disease, and therefore have a skewed, partial perspective of the illness.

Alzheimer's Disease as a Spectrum Disorder

The various subcategories of the Alzheimer's spectrum are defined by biomarkers and clinical symptoms.

Preclinical Alzheimer's

- Individuals with preclinical Alzheimer's have biological markers but no measurable cognitive impairment.

- This stage may last for decades and the person may never develop Alzheimer's.

Mild Cognitive Impairment
- Patients have salient biological markers and have measurable cognitive deficits.
- Some of these patients will stay stable, improve over time, or even ultimately be fine; some will go on to develop clinical Alzheimer's. Brain reserve and cognitive reserve may influence the outcome.
- Patients in this group can sometimes, based on the criteria used and level of functional impairment, be classified as having Alzheimer's.

Alzheimer's Dementia
- Patients with Alzheimer's have biological markers and measurable cognitive deficits that are interfering with function. I subcategorize my patients as follows:

Slowly progressive Alzheimer's disease
- Responsive to treatment.
- Patients are protected against decline by high levels of cognitive and brain reserve.

Rapidly progressive Alzheimer's disease
- More resistant to treatment.

- Patients are not as protected by high levels of cognitive or brain reserve.
- Language, visuospatial, and life skills are affected earlier.

Symptoms and Severity Staging

I assess major symptom categories based on objective neurocognitive testing, including the areas of language, memory, visuospatial ability, and life skills. Each area is then individually rated based on neurocognitive and clinical evaluation to provide nuanced, accurate information. The ratings are excellent, good, mild, moderate, and severe.

JONATHAN'S ALZHEIMER'S DISEASE

As I said earlier, not everyone with early onset has rapidly progressive Alzheimer's. Twenty years ago, while I was at Columbia University's Alzheimer's Center, I met Jonathan, a young man of 44 who worked as an accountant at a law firm. After an extensive workup that included functional PET scans and neurocognitive and laboratory testing, a diagnosis of Alzheimer's was made by our university team, and Jonathan was started on medication. About four years after his diagnosis, he had to stop working and go on disability. His Alzheimer's diagnosis was independently confirmed by other neurolo-

63

gists, as well as several physicians working for his disability insurance firm over the years.

Today, Jonathan is 64. He still comes to see me on his own by subway. His memory is mildly-moderately impaired, and his language and life skills are good. He lives alone with oversight from his longtime girlfriend. He goes to the gym daily, he socializes, and he is compliant with his medication. He could have given up and thrown in the towel, but he didn't. This type of proactive, positive-yet-realistic approach has paid off for Jonathan. It has made it possible for him to now, so many years later, come back from a weekend with his girl-friend in New Orleans with a smile on his face and tell me about it.

MASQUERADING AS ALZHEIMER'S

On occasion, an evaluation of memory loss can lead to surprising results. Sarah's case stands out in my mind, because it underlines the reason for a thorough evaluation rather than simply assuming that the memory loss is from Alzheimer's or another type of de-mentia.

"I've never seen my mother like this. She's been so confused of late," said Sarah's daughter, Lisa, a nurse who worked in the same hospital I did. "Until recently, Mom was up at the crack of dawn and was so put together," she continued. "Even after she retired, she was still out and about, going for walks, taking the dog to the park, going shopping. She was busier than I was, even though I'm the one who's working. Now she is so confused. She's been wetting the sofa she sits on all day, watching TV. Her apartment reeks of urine. I think she has Alzheimer's disease."

Lisa's mother, Sarah, was sitting across from me, looking at me with a little smile on her face. She was overweight, with clear skin and black, gray-flecked hair that she had pulled back into a bun. She was wearing a dress and white nurse's shoes — the type of shoes she'd been comfortable wearing for the forty years that she too had been a nurse, like her daughter was now.

"I don't know what Lisa's saying," Sarah said. "I don't recall wetting the couch. I do feel like I don't have much energy anymore, though. Maybe it has to do with my brain tumor."

Fifteen years earlier, Sarah had had a small brain tumor removed, after which she had undergone some radiation therapy.

Subsequently, she attributed many of her problems to the long-term effects of her brain tumor removal and radiation.

"If she forgets her keys," Lisa said, "it's from the radiation effects. If she gets angry with the grandkids, it's because of the brain tumor. She blames everything on the brain tumor, and now she's saying her behavior lately is because of it too! The brain tumor hasn't come back — we did a scan a couple of months ago to make sure. She is behaving like the dementia patients on my floor."

I listened as Sarah told me about her incontinence, her progressive disorientation, her confusion at times and lucidity at other times. It sounded like rapidly progressing dementia, but something didn't feel quite right.

"How often do you go to the bathroom?" I asked.

"I can't say exactly, but it seems like every other minute," Sarah said.

"Do you drink a lot of water?" I asked.

"Sure, I drink a lot of water." Sarah shrugged. "Isn't that what we're supposed to do? We've got to keep hydrated, right?" she said, ever the nurse.

"Her vitals have been fine," Lisa interjected, guessing correctly that I was looking for medical problems. "I checked her blood pressure the other day and it was perfect. She doesn't have a fever, so I don't think she has an infection."

The wondrous thing about medicine is that when you've trained in it, after a while, all the disparate pieces of a complex puzzle come together at once and punch you in the gut, in a sudden, almost visceral sensation. Sarah's symptoms made sense to me in one of those "aha" moments known to every physician wrestling with diagnostic possibilities.

I got a urine sample from Sarah and tested it. Once I had the results, we discovered the cause of all her problems. Here we were, wondering whether she had residual issues from her long-ago treated brain tumor or whether she was developing dementia, when what Sarah really had was an easily treatable condition: diabetes. Diabetes is generally diagnosed quite easily, but in Sarah's case, her other conditions colluded to make it difficult to uncover. Endocrine disorders, such as diabetes and hypothyroidism, create metabolic changes in the body that can severely affect our cognitive functioning, as they did in Sarah's case.

About Those Plaques

The amyloid plaque deposits that are found in the brains of patients with Alzheimer's disease are not the same plaques found in teeth or in arteries. They are abnormal deposits of a brain protein that are removed from a healthy brain and eliminated, but start accumulating in the brains of those who develop Alzheimer's. These plaques are found in clumps, surrounded by the arms of nerve cells that become distorted near the plaques, likely affected by plaque toxicity.

Some scientists believe the plaques are harmful and lead to cell death, and others believe that the plaques sequester the harmful protein components to prevent cell death.

Some people with plaques have no evidence of memory loss because they are protected by a resilient brain with large cognitive and brain reserves and by unique immune systems that protect them from plaque toxicity.

The Amyvid PET scan for plaque and the spinal tap test for brain plaque and tangles improves diagnostic accuracy in living patients. In the past, plaque could be seen only at autopsy and an Alzheimer's diagnosis could be confirmed only after death.

Scans for abnormal tangles — twisted knots of protein inside nerve cells that disrupt the cell's functioning and cause cell death, another hallmark of Alzheimer's — will soon become commercially available and are even better correlated with clinical symptoms than plaque deposits.

LOOKING FORWARD

Patients on the Alzheimer's spectrum fear the future, because they are faced with the grim prospect of a world that holds little meaning and no joy for them. Fortunately, this is not accurate for most of my patients. I hope that by meeting Bella, Joe, Megan, and Catherine, you have some sense of the functional spectrum that is Alzheimer's. Bella or Joe or Megan could be your co-worker, your neighbor, or your boss, and you wouldn't know they were suffering from Alzheimer's. Patients with Alzheimer's should view themselves and be viewed by others as functional and productive members of their communities — because they generally are.

Most patients live on with a sense of purpose and dignity into old age, especially with early treatment. Therapeutic nihilism is misguided and prevents people who would benefit from treatment from receiving the care they need. Effective treatments are available and should be sought and used to benefit the patient, as we will explore in the next chapter.

CHAPTER 2
I HAVE ALZHEIMER'S: NOW WHAT?
ALZHEIMER'S AS A SPECTRUM DISEASE — AND USING A MULTIPRONGED TREATMENT APPROACH

"I'm not sure why Dr. Franklin sent me to see you," Charles said. "He thought I might have some memory problems, but I haven't really noticed anything."

Charles, who had been referred to me by his internist, was a tall 79-year-old wearing a suit and tie and looking very much like the banker that he was.

As Charles and I talked, I also thought that perhaps Dr. Franklin had been rather quick to send him over. My initial evaluation revealed no evidence that Charles was having any problems. He was still going to work every day and successfully managing multiple funds. Although he had recently acquired a junior partner, his explanation seemed reasonable and not related to cognitive decline. "I'm not going to live forever — I'm getting to that age when I should have someone trained to step in for me," he said.

Although I trusted Dr. Franklin's clinical judgment implicitly, there was nothing in my initial evaluation that made me think that Charles warranted further testing. Charles told me that no one in his family had noticed anything amiss with him. However, to be safe, I called Charles's wife, Alyssa, with his permission.

"I'm calling on behalf of your husband," I said when she answered. "I want to get some information about how his memory's been."

"He's been a little bit more forgetful lately," Alyssa told me, in contrast to Charles's contention that no one at home had noticed a problem. "Does he have Alzheimer's or something?"

"What do you mean by forgetful?" I asked.

"He forgets dates. He used to have a good memory, but now he seems very scattered. I don't know if it's because he's getting older. Does he have Alzheimer's?" she asked again.

Before I could answer, Alyssa said, "So what if he does have Alzheimer's? Even if he does, there's nothing that can be done, right?"

"At this point we don't know whether Charles has Alzheimer's — I'm going to have to do some testing. But I want you to know that there are effective treatments available for the disease if the tests turn out to be positive."

"Really?" Alyssa said, sounding unconvinced.

I sent Charles off for testing, and the results surprised me. His MRI and laboratory tests were normal as I had anticipated, but his memory on neurocognitive testing was profoundly impaired. He scored in the lowest 2 percent for some areas of his memory, compared with other men in his age group, but his overall abilities were far higher. There clearly had been a significant deterioration in his memory, even though he continued to function at a very high level.

At my request, Alyssa came in with Charles for his diagnostic visit. I explained to the two of them that Charles had slowly progressive Alzheimer's, with moderate memory impairment and good language and life skills. (When I use a modifier like *moderate* to describe Charles's memory impairment, I base it on multiple scores from his extensive neurocognitive evaluation, not just his poor second percentile showing in some areas of his memory.)

"Can he still go to work?" Alyssa asked.

"Yes," I said, "he can continue to work."

"But what if people find out about him? What about his judgment?"

"So far he's been good at work," I pointed out. "There have been no complaints, and he's been managing quite well."

"I know. But what about in the future?"

"Unfortunately, we won't know more until he's been treated."

"Yes, I understand," Alyssa said. "But you're telling me that he has Alzheimer's!"

"I would like to do one more test. There's a special scan to see if he has plaque in his brain. If he does, he might be eligible for some studies, which I think would be worthwhile for him, because he has such mild functional impairment and such good cognitive and brain reserve."

"I don't know what that means," Alyssa said, not unreasonably.

"If you think of your brain as a computer," I said, "brain reserve is your hardware — the number of nerve cells you have. If you had a stroke or a brain injury, it would kill some nerve cells and your brain reserve would be reduced. Some people are born with larger brains, just like some computers have more built-in memory. Charles has good brain reserve because he hasn't had a stroke or other brain injury and his MRI showed very little atrophy or shrinkage."

"And cognitive reserve — what's that?"

"Cognitive reserve is your brain's software. It's dependent on the connections between your nerve cells and how quickly and in what way you process information. An active lifestyle, socializing, higher education, and brain exercises make your brain more resilient and increase the connections between your nerve cells. Increasing your cognitive reserve can actually positively loop back to improve your brain reserve by strengthening connections between nerve cells and keeping the cells more active and healthy. Charles has good cognitive reserve because he has a high level of education, plays bridge and golf, and is still working."

"So you're telling me that Charles's condition is treatable?" Alyssa asked skeptically.

"Yes," I said.

But the next day, Alyssa called the office. "I've been reading about Alzheimer's," she said. "There's no cure for it and there are no treatments. I don't know why we would bother doing more tests."

"That's not true," I tried to reassure her again. "There are effective treatments. Each person progresses differently, and many people like Charles, who is still very functional, stabilize with treatment."

"Oh?" she said, still incredulous. "That's

not what I'm reading. That's not what people are telling me."

A few days later, my secretary told me that Alyssa had canceled further testing for Charles, saying, "I don't think anything can help him."

I found this tragic on many levels. If I had told Charles and Alyssa that Charles had cancer and had six months to live, but that with treatment, he would live a year, I would venture to say that Alyssa would have been a lot more proactive and receptive to treatment. But a diagnosis of Alzheimer's often confers a degree of lassitude in the patient and the family, which I believe is counterproductive and harmful. Charles himself did not insist on treatment, because he lacked insight into his condition and did not believe anything was wrong with him.

It is my opinion that with treatment, Charles could have continued to work for a few more years and live a relatively productive life at home. As it is, I have no idea what happened to him.

This reluctance to either investigate or to treat Alzheimer's is prevalent, not just in patients and their families, but also in physicians. As I mentioned earlier, up to 97 percent of mild Alzheimer's cases go undetected in primary care physicians' offices because symptoms are either not noticed or are thought to be part of the normal aging process. The question of what constitutes "normal" in aging depends on the individual's idea of what normal forgetfulness might look like. In addition, 50 percent of moderate Alzheimer's cases go undetected and untreated. In Charles's case, even I, "the dementia expert," was taken in by Charles's togetherness, whereas his astute internist of many years was able to see the changes, as was his wife. Charles's internist could have dismissed his changes as normal for his age, particularly in light of his overall high level of functioning, but wanted to investigate further. Unfortunately for Charles, however, no treatment was started despite his diagnosis of dementia.

How Did Megan Do?

In the last chapter, we met Joe and Bella, who both opted to treat their Alzheimer's aggressively and met with good results; they both continued to work, remained socially engaged, and maintained a good quality of life. We also met Megan, who had just started her treatment. I had predicted that she would respond well despite her relative youth at age 69 and the severity of her plaque deposits, because she had good brain and cognitive reserves. Was that, in fact, the case?

Megan started taking donepezil (Aricept) and memantine (Namenda), two oral medications approved by the Food and Drug Administration to treat Alzheimer's. She also began off-label weekly transcranial magnetic stimulation (TMS) treatments — more on this a little later — as well as weekly tailored, one-on-one brain exercise sessions. Six months later, when tested, Megan had improved significantly across the board on her neurocognitive evaluation, although her memory was still impaired. She also noticed that she was doing better at her job.

A year and a half later, two years after her diagnosis, Megan is stable and continuing to work. She is, finally, as she describes it with a wry smile, "cautiously optimistic." It took two years to convince Megan that her type of Alzheimer's could be successfully treated, but it was well worth it.

Joe and Bella have also done well on a combination of medication, TMS, and brain exercises with some tailored tweaking. Bella, for example, loved her weekly brain exercise programs, but Joe did not take to them and has not continued them. Because Alzheimer's is a spectrum disease — and because every patient is unique — there is no one-size-fits-all treatment. Each person responds differently to treatment, and the choice of regimen depends not only on the type of Alzheimer's disease the patient has but also on the patient's preferences and comfort level.

Treatments for Alzheimer's Disease

I believe in a multipronged approach to treating Alzheimer's and maintaining function, using lifestyle and diet changes to boost overall health as well as both FDA-approved and off-label treatments. I advocate the following:

• Diet modifications to improve health by optimizing caloric intake to achieve an ideal body mass index (BMI) of 24 or lower, and conforming to the American Heart Association diet, which is very similar to the Mediterranean diet

• Treating any medical illnesses such as high blood pressure, diabetes, thyroid dysfunction, and high cholesterol

• Physical exercise, including weight-bearing for bone health and aerobic exercise three days a week

• Improving behavioral health by treating symptoms such as depression, aggression, and anxiety

- Tailoring brain exercises to the individual. For example, someone who has difficulties finding words does exercises to bolster this brain area. These are best done by trained personnel, such as a speech therapist or psychologist. Sudoku, crossword puzzles, and other types of brainteasers can also be helpful for some patients on the Alzheimer's spectrum.

Depending on the patient, I also may prescribe the following medications and treatments:
- Cholinesterase inhibitors such as donepezil (Aricept), galantamine (Razadyne), and rivastigmine (Exelon). These drugs raise levels of the brain chemical acetylcholine, which is present in memory circuits and is reduced in Alzheimer's disease. They come in patch or pill form, with nausea, diarrhea, and dizziness being the most common side effects. Starting at a low dose and slowly increasing it allows most patients to tolerate these drugs. Although the general thinking has been that they cease to work after a few years, I have found them to have utility for many years. Nearly all the patients with Alzheimer's in my practice are on a drug in this class.
- Memantine (Namenda), a drug that works

by reducing toxicity from overactivity of the brain chemical glutamate. The FDA has approved memantine for moderate to severe dementia, but has not found it to be beneficial in mild dementia. I personally have found it to be useful for most patients on the spectrum. When given once a day, in the morning, it is generally well tolerated, with the most common side effect being drowsiness.

- Namzaric, an FDA-approved donepezil-memantine combination. Because it needs to be taken only once a day, it offers ease of use.
- TMS (transcranial magnetic stimulation). TMS is FDA-approved but not for Alzheimer's (for which benefits are unproved).
- Over-the-counter vitamin and dietary supplements, including vitamins E, B_6, B_{12}, D, and folic acid, reservatrol, gingko biloba, omega-3 fish oil, and curcumin. (Benefits are unproved for Alzheimer's.)

I'm also a fan of participating in clinical trials, especially trials using monoclonal antibodies that target plaque deposition in the brain, which seem promising but are still unproved. Up-to-date clinical trial information can be found at clinicaltrials

DEMENTIA: SHE HAS IT; SHE DOESN'T; SHE HAS IT; SHE DOESN'T

Susan was an overweight 87-year-old with high blood pressure and arthritis, whose children brought her in to see me about her severe memory loss. She lived at home with her husband, who was a little older and quite ill. Susan's forgetfulness meant that her blood pressure would often get quite high because she frequently forgot to take her medications.

Susan's memory was poor when I started to see her, so much so that every time I left the room and came back in, she would greet me with a quick laugh and a warm, new "hello!," forgetting that she had seen me just a few minutes before.

After Susan's first visit, an extensive workup was done, and I gave her a diagnosis of slowly progressive Alzheimer's disease with moderate memory and life skills impairment and good language skills, and prescribed donepezil and memantine. However, Susan's internist thought that her memory loss was normal for an 87-year-old woman and that she did not have dementia.

Ambiguity about what constitutes normal can lead to the same patient being diagnosed with dementia by one physician and found to be normal by another. The diagnostic confusion can start with the internist and extend all the way up to "experts" in the dementia field. To make matters more complicated, even when we so-called experts agree that a patient may have dementia, we may disagree about the type of dementia. Susan's children decided to seek a second opinion. They took her to see another physician, a geriatric subspecialist in dementia, who also told them nothing was wrong with their mother.

The children were bewildered, because they knew that their mother's memory had deteriorated dramatically over the previous two years. They did not attribute it simply to old age, because their father, Susan's husband, despite his grave medical issues and being four years older, still had an excellent memory at 91. As a result, Susan's family sought out yet another opinion, this time with a neurologist at a university memory disorder center. Susan was diagnosed with a different type of dementia, Lewy body dementia, not Alzheimer's. I was relieved that she was at least diagnosed with a form of dementia and that her problems weren't merely dismissed as "normal aging." The neurologist at the memory disorder center suggested an approach to treating Susan that was different from mine, which was discussed with her children.

COEXISTING CONDITIONS TO TREAT IN ALZHEIMER'S PATIENTS

Often dementia patients have coexisting medical conditions. Treating these conditions can help maintain cognitive stability. Here are some of the common medical conditions that can coexist with Alzheimer's:

Osteopenia and osteoporosis • Hypertension • High cholesterol • Heart disease • Diabetes • Strokes • Depression • Obesity • Sleep apnea • Insomnia

---

"We're so confused. We don't know what to do," they told me. "You say Mom has Alzheimer's disease, her internist and another doctor say she's fine, and another says she has a dementia but that it isn't Alzheimer's. Whom should we believe? More importantly, how do we treat it?"

This kind of diagnostic confusion is not uncommon in the field. As with other multifaceted medical illnesses, the factors that influence diagnosis and treatment can be complex and the outcome less than clear-cut. Susan's family and I eventually solved the dilemma by agreeing to disagree with the physicians who said she was normal. This left us with the task of deciding on the type of dementia that she had. The definitive test for differentiating between dementia caused by Lewy body disease and that caused by Alzheimer's would be a plaque scan, which Susan refused. As the family opted ultimately to stay under my care and because the treatment approaches to both Alzheimer's and Lewy body are similar, I treated her as someone with Alzheimer's.

Two years into her treatment, Susan has improved dramatically. Recently, she told me a piece of the plot of *Roman Holiday,* one of her (and my) favorite movies, along with the names of two of her (and my) favorite actors: Gregory Peck and Audrey Hepburn. Some of this improvement may be attributed to her agreeing to have her blood pressure and other medications supervised, but in my opinion much of it is due to the treatment of her dementia. Even in cases like Susan's where the diagnosis isn't straightforward, appropriate treatment can be instituted and lead to significant improvement.

MORE DIAGNOSTIC CONFUSION

I diagnosed Vera with slowly progressive Alzheimer's when she was 82, and prescribed memantine and donepezil. Eight years later, Vera had done remarkably well — in fact, her memory had improved. Her two sons began to wonder if she really did have Alzheimer's. They simply did not understand how someone with the disease could stay stable.

"Alzheimer's is different in different people," I explained. "Your mom has responded to treatment and done well."

Nonetheless, the sons decided to seek a second opinion to find out what might be going on with her. The other neurologist did a thorough evaluation and felt that Vera's dementia was more likely related to strokes than to Alzheimer's. However, both Vera's initial MRI from years back and a recent one ordered by the neurologist found no evidence of strokes. Vera's dementia, the neurologist concluded, was, in fact, caused by Alzheimer's.

Vera's was another situation where the family came to understand that the popular narrative of Alzheimer's is inaccurate.

Despite common beliefs to the contrary, with appropriate treatment, people like Vera can stay stable for many years while battling dementia.

I like to think of Alzheimer's as a large iceberg, with most people being aware only of the visible tip — the small proportion of adults with advanced disease — while the vast majority of those who could and should be treated float along, unnoticed. At the risk of being repetitive, keep in mind that between 90 and 97 percent of patients with mild dementia go undiagnosed, even in their internists' offices. This means that only 3 to 10 percent — very much the tip of the Alzheimer's iceberg — of patients get diagnosed, never mind get treatment.

"WATER HEAD" — ALZHEIMER'S COEXISTING WITH OTHER BRAIN DISEASE

Not uncommonly, Alzheimer's disease coexists with other brain disorders that can also impair cognition and can even cause dementia on their own, including strokes and excessive fluid buildup in the brain. Effective treatment must address all conditions for the patient to stay independent. It is also important to aggressively treat medical illnesses, such as high blood pressure, diabetes, and high cholesterol, which, although not primarily brain diseases, nonetheless affect brain health and functioning.

Dr. Peters, a retired psychiatrist, wobbled into my office nearly eight years ago, flanked by his two sons. He couldn't walk straight, and at 73, he was noticing some severe impairment in his memory. He told me, "I can barely take care of myself anymore. Between my memory and my walking, I can't seem to handle things like I used to."

Dr. Peters was divorced and lived alone in an apartment. His sons worried about him being on his own.

"We're thinking we might have to put Dad in a nursing home," one of the sons told me. "He's been falling more and he's been confused. We are worried he might fall at home and no one will know. We call him daily, but still . . ."

"Not so fast," I said. "Let's see what we can do for him."

One of the first things I wanted to do was a spinal tap, because I thought that Dr. Peters's memory loss might be related to an excess of fluid buildup in the brain — a condition called *hydrocephalus,* a word that literally means "water brain/head." I thought that might be why he was having trouble with his walking.

"Oh, no!" the sons exclaimed, when they heard about the spinal tap. "That sounds pretty dangerous."

But Dr. Peters reassured his sons. "I did many spinal taps on patients when I was younger. It's really quite safe, and you shouldn't worry about it."

His sons agreed to the spinal tap, and mere days after the procedure, Dr. Peters improved dramatically. He no longer tee-tered like someone who had had way too much alcohol or had just stepped off a boat. Instead, he was able to walk confidently without assistance. This confirmed my thinking that pressure from excess cerebro-spinal brain fluid had been causing his symptoms.

Given the unquestionable improvement after the excess cerebrospinal fluid drainage via the spinal tap, I arranged for Dr. Peters to have a ventriculo-peritoneal shunt placed. This involved the insertion of a small tube to drain fluid from his blocked brain cavi-ties into his abdominal cavity, where it was reabsorbed into circulation. Although the procedure may sound scary, it is in fact relatively simple with a low complication rate, and patients go home a day or two after surgery.

Dr. Peters's walking improved dramatically after the operation, but his memory remained poor. I diagnosed him with slowly progressive Alzheimer's with mild memory loss and no language or life skills impairment, in addition to his hydrocephalus. I started him on donepezil and memantine, and added an antidepressant for his low-level depression. Dr. Peters responded well and was able to live alone and take care of himself for six years.

At that point his memory had deteriorated to the point that he was forgetting to take his medications and did not seem to be eating well. Understanding he could no longer cope entirely on his own, his sons made arrangements for an aide to go into their father's home for a few hours each day to help him with activities like bathing, shopping, and cooking. This caregiver was also able to offer their father companionship, something he sorely needed. He initially fought the arrangement tooth and nail, but once he met his new caregiver, Dr. Peters changed his mind. The two of them took to each other and went out for lunch every day.

Thanks to this additional help, we avoided putting him in a nursing home. His sons and I were proud that Dr. Peters continued to live in his own home and was able to walk unassisted, until he died in his sleep, in his own bed, at 82.

Dr. Peters is a good example of how being proactive about treatment — including treating coexisting medical issues — can help maintain a patient's quality of life and allow them to stay in their own home.

SEEKING CREATIVE SOLUTIONS

Sometimes, appropriate and affordable treatment of patients with dementia requires thinking outside the box.

My 77-year-old patient Chloe, a retired teacher from the Fashion Institute of Technology with a fondness for wearing couture clothing, came in on her own for a memory assessment. I diagnosed her with slowly progressive Alzheimer's disease with mild memory loss, moderate language impairment, and good life skills. She was still living alone and seemed to be managing well. However, upon hearing her diagnosis, her two children, who both lived in faraway states, decided that their only option was to place their mom in a nursing home.

"You have to help me, Dr. Devi," Chloe said. "My daughters want to put me away. I've tried to convince them that I'm fine where I am, but they are hell-bent on getting me into one of these old folks' homes, and I really don't want that."

With Chloe's permission, I arranged for a conference call with her two children.

"She'll be safer here and closer to me," said one of Chloe's daughters. "There's a great place right down the street, and she'll be closer to her grandchildren." This is a common reason for moving patients with dementia: the well-intentioned "closer to me" rationalization. The problem is that from the patient's perspective, they are being uprooted, taken away from their friends, routines, and home to live in a strange place, albeit closer to a loved one.

"But we haven't even begun to treat her yet," I implored, advocating on behalf of Chloe. "Let's treat her and see how she responds."

They agreed, but a problem remained: how to get Chloe to take her medications. She often forgot to do so, despite her best intentions. One of her daughters agreed to call and remind her, but even so, Chloe would forget her pills. I decided that she needed someone to visit her once a day, even if for a half hour, to physically supervise her taking her medications. Chloe's daughters were able to get a neighbor to perform this task for a small payment.

Chloe has responded well to her treatment. She has continued to live at home, independently, for the five years since we first met. This little tweak — finding a neighbor who was willing and able to help for a short time daily — helped Chloe maintain her independence.

I should add that I do my best to enable my patients to take their medications just once a day. I coordinate with their other physicians, and if some medications require multiple doses a day, we either substitute a different medication or consolidate dosages. In about three quarters of my patients, I am able to achieve a once-daily medication regimen, which improves compliance in general and streamlines external help in situations like Chloe's.

TRANSCRANIAL BRAIN STIMULATION
Dr. Smith, a retired 86-year-old internist, was sent to me by his own internist for a second opinion on treatment options. The year before, Dr. Smith had been given a diagnosis of Alzheimer's by another neurologist, who had inexplicably decided not to treat him. When I asked Dr. Smith about it, he said that the neurologist thought treatment would not help. Despite misgivings, Dr. Smith had not questioned the decision, but as he continued to decline, he had

complained to his internist, which had prompted this visit. By the time I saw him, Dr. Smith had had memory loss for three years. After testing, I diagnosed him with slowly progressive Alzheimer's disease with moderate memory and language loss and good life skills.

I started him on oral medications, and then we discussed a course of off-label treatment with transcranial magnetic stimulation (TMS). TMS is FDA-approved for treating depression and a specific type of migraine. I have spent a decade investigating the effects of TMS in patients with Alzheimer's and thought it would help Dr. Smith significantly, especially with his failing language skills. Remember the concept of brain reserve and cognitive reserve? TMS increases cognitive reserve by increasing connections in targeted neural circuits. With TMS treatment, a magnetic field from a table-tennis-sized paddle held against the scalp changes brain activity in a penny-sized area of brain under the paddle, while patients sit, watch television, or read. It can also increase brain reserve, although it does so less robustly. TMS will likely be approved for stroke rehabilitation in the near future because of its ability to both reduce recovery time and increase functional gain. European data shows strong evidence for its utility in treating chronic pain that is resistant to medications, and I have found this to be true as well.

A large trial is taking place using TMS to treat Alzheimer's because of promising results from earlier trials, including my own. TMS has helped many of my Alzheimer's patients with their language, motor, and life skills. In my experience, about 20 percent of patients improve with TMS treatment, and another 40 percent stay stable, but other researchers have found improvements in up to 80 percent of patients. These changes are caused by the engagement of specific circuits, leading to new neural pathway growth, a process known as neuroplasticity.

Dr. Smith thrived with TMS and his medications. He had also started weekly one-on-one brain exercises, which he found helpful. Unfortunately, because of the cost of TMS treatment — which insurance did not cover because it was off-label — his family decided to discontinue his regimen abruptly after a year and a half. I had developed a great fondness for Dr. Smith, and by the time he was removed from my care, he and I had established a high level of rapport and respect for each other. I did not have a chance to say goodbye to Dr. Smith, which saddened me.

About two weeks later, my secretary buzzed me. "I have Dr. Smith on the phone for you," she said.

"Dr. Devi, I'm sorry I didn't have a chance to say goodbye," he told me. "I want to tell you how grateful I am for all your help. Before I saw you, I had been told nothing could be done for me, but you helped me, so thank you."

On the one hand the conversation made me happy — I was glad that Dr. Smith's memory had improved to the point where he was able to remember my number and make the call, things he had had difficulty doing before he came to see me. I was also happy that I was able to be of some assistance to him. But the call also made me sad. Dr. Smith would no longer be getting the help that he needed to maintain his improvements.

In an illness like stroke, where there is a "one-time" destruction, brain stimulation is no longer needed after brain function is recovered. With an illness like Alzheimer's, however, where there is continued assault on the brain by newly forming deposits of plaques and tangles, ongoing treatment is needed. That said, in my research we found that even just four sessions of TMS appeared to maintain increased blood flow in the neural circuitry on functional MRI scanning for as long as a month after stopping treatment, and possibly for longer. Dr. Smith likely maintained the benefits obtained from TMS for at least a few months, if not more, after ceasing treatment.

WHEN PAIN MASKS ALZHEIMER'S

Another patient, Ellis, was 82 when I first saw him for severe intractable pain of unknown origin that left him screaming for hours every day. Although much of my research and clinical focus has been in the area of memory loss, I, like other neurologists, also treat patients with conditions like chronic pain, migraines, seizures, and strokes. Because Ellis moaned throughout the visit, barely participating in the examination, I got his history from his wife, Barbara. He had seen several physicians and not found any relief. I placed Ellis on a regimen of nonaddictive pain medication, and he improved to the point where he barely noticed any discomfort. However, he continued to use a walker and seemed disinclined to walk, which puzzled me. It reminded me of patients with dementia who don't recover as they should after a medical illness.

97

About two months after he first came to see me, Ellis was no longer in pain and was able to cooperate with a proper examination. I discovered that Ellis's memory was not what it should be. Both his wife and I had focused on his pain and not noticed his cognition deficits. Ellis had a thorough cognitive evaluation, including an Amyvid plaque scan. I diagnosed him with rapidly progressive Alzheimer's with moderate memory, language, and life skills impairment.

I prescribed medication for his memory and had him begin physical therapy to try to wean him off his walker, but he was not able to give it up. After two months of this, I prescribed a course of targeted TMS sessions for Ellis. I wasn't sure that it would help, given the severity of his condition, but within a month, he was able to get around without his walker. He began to interact more fully with his family, and I got a sense of his personality, including his sardonic sense of humor. After completing a year of treatment, he even took trips as far away as Australia and New Zealand. It was a dramatic improvement that many naysayers would consider impossible.

Because of the expensive equipment and staff needed, TMS remains a higher-cost option. Once a particular treatment is approved for a particular condition, insurance companies are charged with covering the costs. Because TMS is now approved in the United States for treating depression, insurance companies have instituted coverage for this diagnosis. Although TMS is not yet approved in the United States for treating Alzheimer's, stroke, or chronic pain, there is a growing body of research speaking to the utility of this treatment for these conditions, consistent with my own research and clinical experience.

BRAIN EXERCISES

The brain is an organ that embraces the concept of "learned nonuse." The less you use a certain part of the brain, the less likely you are to use it over time, the fewer connections in that circuit, and the more difficult it becomes to access. Grandma was right when she said, "Use it or lose it."

When dementia patients have trouble with language, for example, they will often withdraw into themselves, and their world literally gets quieter as a result. With that quietness, the patients' functioning becomes worse and they lose even more of their ability to speak. This neuroplasticity, both positive and negative, is ongoing in all of us.

For example, try swearing when you're frustrated for even a week and you will find that it becomes almost automatic. Stop for a few weeks and then try a swear word — it is more difficult to access and harder to let roll off the tongue. Whereas TMS modulates neural circuitry even in uncooperative patients, one-on-one brain exercises offer similar benefits to patients like Megan who want to participate actively in their care.

When I first began to specialize in dementias in 1994, I was surprised to find that, unlike in patients with stroke or other neurologic disorders, patients with dementia did not receive any targeted behavioral treatments. A stroke patient who had trouble speaking would receive speech therapy. One who had trouble walking would receive physical therapy. Dementia patients with conceptual or language problems received no such care. When I started my memory center in 1999, I began to focus on this neglected area with my dementia patients. It made no neurobiological sense to me that we would give up on activating brain regions just because a patient had a dementia diagnosis. Patients may be forgetful, I thought, but in many cases — at least in my practice — they were still cognitively competent in other areas. It seemed tragic to write them off.

I reasoned that cognitive remediation, a sort of "physical therapy for the brain," might help. I designed a program of cognitive exercises for my patients with Alzheimer's that they would do, under supervision, in my office once or twice a week. I found that this helped patients maintain their level of functioning. Many patients enjoyed having cognitive "homework" to do. It also affected their outlook on the illness — they felt they could do something to stave off decline, rather than simply sitting and waiting for the illness to progress.

I divided the exercises into categories: language and comprehension, verbal and visual memory, visuospatial skills, and abstract thinking. For example, if a patient was having trouble with language, we would go through a series of structured cognitive exercises designed to help her maintain access to words. These routines helped prevent decline and preserved the ability to speak fluently, read, and write. Such skills can be lost if they are not used regularly, and maintaining them allows a person to continue participating fully in life. This, of course, has a significant effect on one's sense of well-being.

I remember being looked at askance by

101

some colleagues back in 1999 for my belief in the benefits of cognitive exercises in patients with dementia. The conventional wisdom at that time was that cognitive exercises would not work or make any discernible difference in patients with Alzheimer's. Since then, numerous studies have shown that brain exercises do, in fact, have a place in the care of patients with Alzheimer's. Some health insurance companies have also started to cover these treatments for patients with dementia.

I continue to strongly believe that cognitive remediation improves daily living skills, attention, and language, and that it reduces depression, among other benefits. Even so, the perception of physicians and the public remains, for the most part, less positive about the value of such interventions.

NO LONGER A "VEGETABLE"

Mark was an early patient who sealed my belief in the efficacy of brain exercises. He was a 69-year-old retired businessman when I first met him. At the time I was at Columbia University's Alzheimer's Center, where diagnoses were made at a consensus conference by a team of neurologists, psychiatrists, geriatricians, neuropsychologists, and social workers. Mark was diagnosed with Alzheimer's disease. Today, with my view of Alzheimer's as a spectrum disorder, I would refine that diagnosis to slowly progressive Alzheimer's disease, with mild-moderate memory impairment and good language and life skills. He was started on donepezil, and, when it became available, memantine.

Many months after I diagnosed Mark, I left Columbia to start my private practice and he chose to follow me there. We began doing weekly brain exercises, focusing on the areas he was having trouble with, including word finding, attention, and visuospatial function. At that time, I oversaw the exercises myself; now I have wonderfully talented psychologists who have taken over. I enjoyed working with Mark, and he did very well. Five years later, in 2002, when the British Broadcasting Service — the BBC — interviewed me for a program on brain repair, Mark and his wife of fifty years, Brenda, volunteered to speak about their experiences.

Here is the transcript of the broadcast, slightly edited for clarity.

BBC Interviewer: What sort of things do you do with Dr. Devi when you come here?

Mark: All sorts of mental gyrations —

games, I call them — things to stimulate the nerve endings. I was a vegetable before, and now I've learned how to read again, how to write again.

Interviewer: Vegetable is quite a harsh term. Things were that bad?

Mark: Yeah, well, I was unable to read — a very important thing to me. I was unable to do anything with my hands, also very important to me — like artwork, photography, and carpentry, all of which Dr. Devi brought back into my life. I was able to read the newspaper again, which I had forgotten about, as if they never existed.

The interviewer also asked Mark's wife, Brenda, what it was like being a very involved witness in this process.

Brenda: Mark was a world traveler, businessman, active physically and mentally. Then there was lack of interest. Part of it was depression, a sense of diminishment. He realized he was not the same person; he was losing his life. I felt like I was losing my partner — I don't feel that anymore. Now he follows TV, music, art, movies; he's aware and interested in what's going on in the world. We can travel, enjoy theater and movies, and interacting. It's come back in terms of a good quality of life. The prognosis was that he was going to lose it, and instead he's gotten back what he lost. We keep joking, is the diagnosis correct? It was not supposed to work this way.

Mark lived another eight years after this interview and stayed mostly stable, going on cruises with Brenda until the last two years of his life, when he began to deteriorate. We then got him live-in care and he died at home, in comfort, still talking and able to recognize his loved ones.

Diet and Physical Exercise

Improving diet can play a major role in treating patients. Almost any diet that is healthy for the heart is also going to be healthy for the brain. I recommend one that's as close to a Mediterranean diet as possible — high in vegetable content, but also including healthful servings of lean meat, fish, and unsaturated fats like olive oil. The American Heart Association diet is a good one to follow. If patients are overweight, I refer them to nutritionists who work with them to get to a healthier weight.

Patients will often ask me if they are still allowed to have a glass of wine with dinner, and my answer is usually a resounding yes. I feel that the complete prohibition of alcohol isn't necessary. Moderation of intake, on the other hand, is quite another story. I usually advise patients not to drink more than the equivalent of two glasses of wine a day.

I also advise patients to participate in aerobic exercise three days a week, for at least 30 minutes a session, and to do weight-bearing exercises twice a week to maintain their bones. Aerobic exercise increases blood flow to the brain, thus improving cognition, strengthening connections between nerve cells, and boosting cognitive reserve. If patients have balance problems and have either stopped walking or are walking less, I investigate and treat the problems so that their confidence in walking can be restored. If balance continues to be an issue, I have patients use walking poles — similar to ski poles — instead of canes or walkers. These poles can be used rhythmically and promote an upright, natural posture and ergonomic movement. What's more, they convey a sense of health, rather than infirmity.

These relatively simple, inexpensive, and easy-to-implement dietary and exercise interventions have had a significant positive impact on the lives of my patients. Such changes can be adopted not only by those on the clinical end of the Alzheimer's spectrum, but also by those in the "preclinical" stages, before symptoms become apparent. Adopting these lifestyle modifications helps to keep the brain resilient from plaque-driven brain cell loss and can have an enormous effect on a patient's level of functioning.

PROACTIVE PREVENTION

As we near the end of this chapter, I have one final story to share with you. Geraldine was a brisk, no-nonsense 79-year-old who lived alone and came in to see if there was anything she could do to keep from developing Alzheimer's. When she arrived for her appointment, she placed a pile of autopsy reports on my table.

"My father and my aunt both had Alzheimer's disease confirmed at autopsy. Their mother — my grandmother — had it too," she said. "I occasionally forget things, and when I do, I go off the deep end. I'll have a thought in my head, and then I lose it and I go nuts."

Although Geraldine suspected that her forgetting was normal for her age, her family history was hanging over her head.

"Every time I leave my keys behind, I think it's the first sign of Alzheimer's," she said. "I know everyone forgets their keys sometimes, but they don't have a history like mine. If there's a medicine I can take that will push the disease back," she added, pushing the air away with her palm for emphasis, "maybe I will get Alzheimer's later than my father. He called my brother and me 'darling' and 'sweetheart' in the last year of life because he couldn't remember our names.

"My sister said I am out of my mind," she continued. "She told me that if I'm going to get Alzheimer's, then I am and that's it! But I want to do it on my terms — I want to fight this. You've got to get me to age ninety compos mentis, that's my aim."

I admired Geraldine for her determination, her courage and spirit, and her resolve to face the proverbial dragon of her fears. Testing revealed that Geraldine had the E4 type of the APOE gene, moderate plaques on her Amyvid brain scan, minimal memory loss, and evidence of a few strokes. Geraldine turned out to have preclinical Alzheimer's on the spectrum. We began a program of lifestyle modifications, brain exercises, and stroke prevention to help her maintain her level of cognitive function and prevent her from developing symptoms of Alzheimer's.

My story with Geraldine is just starting, so I cannot tell you the ending, but I will say this: I wish more people approached their memory loss concerns the way she did. Because she has the right attitude, I believe we will get her where she wants to be — 90 years old and still in good mental shape.

Because Alzheimer's is a spectrum disease and each patient is unique, a multipronged approach to treatment is essential. It's also important to get a diagnosis and begin treatment early. By using a combination of medications (those already approved and those that show promise), exercises (physical and cognitive), and diet and lifestyle modifications, and by treating coexisting conditions, the patient and the family may enjoy significant benefits. Bella, Joe, Megan, and Mark are proof of the long-term benefits associated with treatment, specifically for the patient but also for society at large, which can continue to enjoy the many contributions that these individuals keep making.

CHAPTER 3
WHETHER I HAVE ALZHEIMER'S DISEASE IS NOBODY'S BUSINESS BUT MY OWN.
WHEN AND HOW TO SHARE THE DIAGNOSIS

I met Ruth at a dinner party for eight. She was elegantly dressed but severe looking, with a sharp, withering glare — the kind of woman whose wrinkles had hardened in all the wrong places. You could imagine her prodding people along with the sharp end of a long, tapered umbrella. Her husband had informed me some time before the dinner that his wife suffered from Alzheimer's, and thanks to him, everyone else at the table had known about Ruth's diagnosis for years. I was seated next to her and tried to draw her into a conversation. But Ruth demurred, rebuffing all my attempts and staring off into the space in front of her, clearly not wanting to be involved.

Eventually, I gave up and conversed with the others at the table. We ended up talking around Ruth, as if she didn't really exist. We were like a sea that ebbed and flowed around the rock that was Ruth, making room for her and oblivious to her at the same time. Every once in a while, someone would ask Ruth a question but not wait for a response, or if they did, they would listen absently, their mind already drifting away. Ruth, with her curt, withdrawn replies and her icy glare, did little to help her cause.

About six months later, her husband called to ask if I would evaluate Ruth because he thought she needed a new doctor. I agreed to see her. I learned from him that since the diagnosis had been made five years earlier, things had changed in unimaginable ways for both of them. Ruth's husband had begun to view her differently. He had become more solicitous of her, and she, in turn, had become more dependent. He asked little of her for fear it would be "too much," and she responded by doing less, all but stopping any housekeeping or socializing. She spoke rarely and mostly spent her waking hours at home, idle and listless. Her husband's description fit with my memories of the unengaged, distant woman at the dinner.

The second time I met Ruth, she was in my waiting room, wearing a boxy suit that succeeded in emphasizing both the hardness and the smallness of her person. I shook her hand, introducing myself as I ushered her into my office.

"You know," she said, "we've met before. I don't know if you recall, but you were sitting next to me at that dinner at Sophia's for Alison's birthday. I remember you wore a beautiful coral sweater."

I hid my surprise. Here was a woman who had been diagnosed with Alzheimer's disease five years earlier, recalling small details that I had forgotten. She had barely spoken and had seemed detached during that dinner, and now she was not only remembering vividly, but also giving me a compliment.

We chatted a little in this social vein, discussing the people at the dinner party — she was able to remember them all. She mentioned parts of the conversation from that evening, including a lengthy discussion about a chicken casserole.

"I think not more than two minutes should be allowed for a conversation on chicken casserole," Ruth said, in an unexpected flash of humor.

I realized in that moment that Ruth had been misdiagnosed with Alzheimer's disease. She didn't even have much of a cognitive problem. In fact, several minutes into her visit, Ruth's memory appeared superior to most.

After a physical and cognitive examination, I discovered that Ruth suffered from mild Parkinson's disease, without any evidence of dementia. Unfortunately, because she had been given a diagnosis of Alzheimer's, everyone around her had been treating her differently for years. Ruth was an inherently proud woman and very concerned about her social persona. She began to respond and react differently because of this sensitivity, and in the end, she began to exhibit behaviors seen in people with dementia. She withdrew and avoided social situations that could be potentially embarrassing. This was a case of life imitating diagnosis.

LOSING THE PERSON FOR THE DISEASE

Although Ruth's case is an extreme example because she was misdiagnosed, her situation shows what can happen when people are told that a friend or a peer has dementia. Few of us would be knowingly unkind or cruel, but as human beings we respond instinctively, labeling people as friend or foe, as smart or slow. When we put a person into the Alzheimer's patient category, rather than thinking, *This is my smart and funny friend Ruth, one of the most interesting people I know,* we may lose the person for the disease. It's easy to start making erroneous assumptions, such as "she's different now," "she's no longer competent," or "I'm not sure she'll understand what I'm saying, so let me talk loudly/simply/slowly/not at all when I'm with her."

Often people don't know how to respond. A patient once told me, "It is really surprising what people say. Not, 'I'm so sorry about what's happening to you,' but rather, 'Oh my God, *I* couldn't exist with Alzheimer's!' As if I had a choice in the matter." Unfortunately, she's not alone in receiving distaste rather than sympathy and understanding from the people in her circle who knew of her diagnosis.

Because of this human tendency to categorize and simplify, and because a diagnosis of Alzheimer's lends itself to all manner of stigmatizing classifications, my usual counsel to patients and their families is "Don't tell." This works much of the time and fails spectacularly on other occasions, because with Alzheimer's, as with most things in life, there is no one-size-fits-all solution. Ultimately, every patient and every family is different, each wrestling with the diagnosis in their own particular way.

HER PERSONALITY?
OR THE DISEASE?

Harold was a short, slender man of 76 with round, wire-rimmed glasses, a balding head, and a fondness for rumpled shirts and cardigans. In other words, he looked every bit like the erudite professor that he was. His wife, Miriam, was 74 with blonde hair, high cheekbones, and a love of unusual earrings and shoes. She had the kind of perfectly coiffed confidence that only someone born beautiful could pull off. Miriam often announced that she had not thought herself the marrying kind until she met Harold in her late thirties.

Miriam was a rather scattered person, and she endearingly admitted to approaching life in an unstructured way. "It's worked like a charm for me," she said. "Everyone else helps out and pinch-hits when I need it."

Harold, on the other hand, prided himself on his organizational abilities, and this odd-couple dance had worked well for both of them for the forty-plus years of their marriage. Lately, however, Miriam's increasing disorganization had Harold concerned.

"Miriam has always been ditzy," Harold said. "But now, she's become — how shall I put this? — über-ditzy. I have to remind her about all her appointments. She forgets more than she ever has."

"Pshaw," Miriam scoffed while gently laughing at Harold. "There's nothing wrong with me. Harold likes things a little too all together, if you ask me. And I find that rather b-o-r-i-n-g. Can you imagine anything more exciting than finding a darling pair of shoes in your closet that you forgot you had? And there are some things I never forget. Ask me about the jewelry I am wearing today. Go ahead, ask me!"

"Tell me about your earrings," I said.

"I am wearing the art deco ones that Harold's mother gave me when we got married. I don't wear them often because they are so valuable, but if coming to see you is not a special occasion, what is?" She flashed me one of her radiant smiles, flushed with triumph. "Did I tell you," she continued, "that I never thought I would marry until I met Harry?"

"She doesn't forget jewelry," Harold said grudgingly. "But ask her what we did yesterday."

Harold was right. Miriam did indeed have trouble remembering what she had done yesterday and what she had had for breakfast. After a series of tests, I discovered that Miriam had rapidly progressive Alzheimer's disease with moderate memory impairment and mild language and life skills impairment. I sat them both down at the diagnostic visit to give them her results. Miriam took the news in with aplomb.

"Okay, so I have Alzheimer's. Tell me what to do," she said.

I told her and Harold how we needed to proceed with treatment — oral medications, TMS, and brain exercises.

"All right," she said, "if you say so. I personally don't think there is anything wrong with me, but I trust you know what you are doing."

Harold, on the other hand, was completely devastated. He had suspected that she was developing Alzheimer's, and now his worst fears were realized. A planner who did his best to control their future, he felt their world was upended. He was now in uncertain territory with Miriam, and neither knew what the future held.

In his panic after being told of the diagnosis, Harold lost sight of a crucial distinction: Each time Miriam was disorganized, there were two possible reasons. One was that it was her inherent "Miriamness." The other was that it was because of the Alzheimer's. Harold became alarmed every time Miriam forgot something, assuming each instance was a sign that her Alzheimer's was getting worse.

"But I've always forgotten things, Harry!" Miriam exclaimed in desperation in my office a few months later. "Okay, maybe I am forgetting more. But I have never had a memory like yours. I never wanted to. It would make me so anxious to remember everything like you do."

Then she turned to me and told me, as she would many times over, "I never wanted to marry until I met Harry. He was the man for me. Even if he never forgets things." Repeating things is a common symptom of Alzheimer's — one that can exasperate family members and caregivers, who may hear the same piece of information or get asked the same question, sometimes literally dozens of times a day. Repetition occurs because some patients lose the ability to store and retrieve more recent memories, so they forget they've told a story or asked a question just a few minutes before.

Despite Miriam's pleas and my attempts to reassure Harold that Miriam's illness would take time to progress, it became exhausting for both Miriam and me to try to calm him down.

He began to hover over her. He started to try to teach her things like maintaining an appointment book and keeping lists — things Miriam had never done in her life. He grew furious because Miriam didn't seem to understand his perspective that organization was the key to helping her forget less. I believe that in his mind, Harold saw organization as a way of vanquishing the illness and keeping it at bay.

"I don't get it!" he said in frustration. "She keeps insisting she is the same. But she is different. She has Alzheimer's, and when I point it out to her, she denies she has it."

"Harold," I said, "Miriam is Miriam. She is mostly the same as she ever was, and also a little different, in that she is even more forgetful. She is not suddenly going to become an organized person. She's spent her whole life laid-back and scattered. She may not dwell on the fact that she has Alzheimer's or that she forgets things. She may choose to describe it as being less organized. But she has been accepting and following the prescribed treatment."

"I know," Harold said, "but wouldn't it be easier if she agreed that she had Alzheimer's? Why does she deny it? Also, I don't see why she can't write things down so she can remember them! I don't see why you can't tell her to do that."

He was getting angry with me, with what he saw as my insensitive approach.

"It's my guess that you deal with stress by becoming even more organized as a way to keep your life sane," I said. "You have to realize that by trying to impose your organization on Miriam, you're only going to make matters more difficult for both of you. I can tell her to write things down and she will forget that I did. Even if she were to write things down, she would misplace the piece of paper, not remember she wrote it down, not remember what she wrote down or where she put it. . . . Your solution seems simple, but it won't work with her, and it'll only make you angrier and more frustrated. It will stress you both out."

I made no headway with Harold, who was getting more enraged by the minute. His anger came from his fear — of losing his wife, their hopes and plans for the future, and their way of life.

Harold was also terrified for another reason. He and Miriam were very social people with a large circle of friends and dined out almost every night. Both he and Miriam agreed that the fewer people who knew of the diagnosis, the better. They believed it was their business and no one else's. While Miriam was fully confident of herself in social situations, Harold now became tense whenever they went out. He was worried that Miriam was going to make a mistake that would reveal her diagnosis to their friends. He spent such evenings sitting by Miriam's side, listening with one ear to what she was saying and using the other for his own conversation. Whenever he felt she was floundering, he'd jump in to quickly correct and fill in for her. In other words, he was completely unable to relax and enjoy himself when they were with company.

Miriam, however, sailed through her lapses, a gilded ship gliding through calm seas. If she forgot a name, she would substitute with a "darling," a "handsome," or a "dear."

"No one even notices," Miriam told me. "I have never been known for my great memory. I have been trying to tell Harry that most people are too self-involved to really care what the other person is saying anyway, but it's very hard for him to understand. He's such a perfectionist."

From my perspective, Miriam was right in her social approach. If someone generally behaves appropriately, the threshold for suspicion of memory loss tends to stay low. If a patient sticks to their "cocktail-party personality" — if they keep conversation light and limited to small talk — it's unusual for others to notice anything amiss.

But the "don't tell" approach was trying on Harold. He was afraid that someone would *discover their secret.* He became more and more anxious with what he felt was the concealment of the elephant in the room. To his credit, he wanted to honor Miriam's wishes regarding her medical privacy. Even so, he could not understand how anyone would fail to notice that she was different.

Miriam, meanwhile, kept insisting, "I keep telling Harold I am the same person, but he keeps saying that I'm changed. Maybe I'm different, but I feel the same to me!" These proclamations only added to Harold's sense of consternation.

Their arguments would erupt in my office at times.

"But you are different!" Harold would insist. "You repeat things. You can't remember our friends' names. You can't cook the way you used to!"

"So I'm a little forgetful. But I'm still me!" Miriam would respond.

Harold and Miriam and Ruth and her

husband give us a sense of what happens when the label "Alzheimer's disease" is applied to a person. It can change the person's perception of themselves, as it did with Ruth. And it can certainly alter others' perception of the person. Both Miriam's and Ruth's husbands' changed in their behavior toward their wives, Ruth's more drastically than Miriam's.

"Alzheimer's is not like the measles," I recall a wise woman telling me once. "You can't see it. It's a behavioral problem and the behavior has to be really obvious for people to notice. If your mom asked you, 'Who are you?' that would be obvious and you'd likely notice. But most people make up explanations for behaviors, like 'maybe my mom was joking.' It is the same with Alzheimer's. If you stay relaxed, most people don't suspect or make excuses on your behalf." She was right, and Miriam knew this intuitively.

JUST DOWN THE STREET

Even I, a specialist in dementia, once failed to notice memory loss when it stared me in the face, cloaked as it was in a social context.

When my daughter, Ginny, was about eight years old, she and I went to a grocery store a few blocks from our home where she met a very nice elderly man in the ice cream section. They struck up a conversation on the relative merits of cookie dough ice cream — Ginny's favorite flavor at the time.

We three ended up in the checkout line together, and the man asked us where we lived.

"Just down the street," I said.

"I live in that direction too," he said, so we started walking back together. After we'd walked about a block, he asked, "Where do you live?"

I repeated, "We live down the street."

Then a couple of blocks later, he asked again: "So, where do you live?"

Once again, I responded, "Just down this street."

This question peppered our conversation, which was about many other things, including the noisiness of New York City; the weather in Kansas, where he was from; and that he was visiting his daughter, who had just had a baby.

As we said our goodbyes, he again asked, "Do you live around here?"

Once more, I said, "Yes, we live down the street."

After we parted ways with the gentleman,

I remarked to Ginny what a nice man he was. "He did talk a lot, though, didn't he?"

She looked at me in surprise and said, "Mom, he was talking a lot because he was repeating himself. He has Alzheimer's disease!"

It was an "A-ha!" moment. I realized immediately that my little daughter was right — our new acquaintance had a memory problem. I had just *failed to notice* and had instead made up an excuse for him, thinking him garrulous instead of forgetful. Children, not as versed in the nuances of social niceties, may sometimes pick up on such problems faster than adults. They notice without passing judgment. If I'd perceived our new friend's repetitions, I might have been more dismissive of him. I hope I wouldn't have, but it's hard to know with human nature. Ginny was aware of our new friend's memory loss, but didn't hesitate to carry on an engrossing conversation with him.

WHEN TO TELL

When a person's memory loss progresses to a point where it seems apparent to all, the "don't tell" policy may no longer seem appropriate. Nonetheless, the patient may still opt to not tell for reasons of privacy and pride. These are important concerns for the patient, and even if the physician or caregiver thinks that the diagnosis is now obvious to most observers and should be made public, I prefer to respect and abide by the patient's wishes. Patients should tell others only if and when they are ready to. Some may choose never to publicly discuss their condition, just as someone with cancer may choose to keep their illness private until their death. Honoring these wishes is essential for the well-being of the person; their preferences shouldn't be dismissed just because they suffer from dementia.

Telling Others
Here are some things to consider when deciding whether to tell people about your Alzheimer's (or dementia) diagnosis.

- People may not understand that Alzheimer's is a spectrum disorder and that it can manifest in many different ways. People may underestimate your competence and intelligence and treat you in ways you find patronizing.
- Your reactions and decisions may be second-guessed and attributed to dementia, even by well-meaning friends and family.
- If your friends and family treat you differ-

126

ently, your confidence may diminish and your anxiety level may rise. As a result, you may be tempted to shun social situations.

All that said, for some people, telling may be better than dealing with the anxiety of keeping the diagnosis private.

CHOOSING NOT TO TELL

Lois, a precise, proper, and fiercely proud retired English teacher, came to see me with her husband, Saul, who had been an actuary and dealt with numbers all day long before he retired. Both were no taller than five foot four. Lois, now in her seventies, was twelve years younger than Saul, who was well into his eighties. They had married when she was 17 and he was 29, and had shared a full life. Their three kids adored them and lived close by, and they enjoyed spending time with their many grandchildren.

Their eldest daughter, Carrie, sent me an email in advance of her mother's visit.

"I think Mom has Alzheimer's. She's very forgetful and it's getting worse day by day. She doesn't see it, though, and my father is forever covering up for her," she wrote. Carrie requested that I not mention to her parents that she had been in touch with me. She knew Lois would be mortified if she realized that Carrie had noticed her forgetfulness. She got Lois to come to see me by surreptitiously reaching out to Lois's internist, who in turn had sent Lois on to me.

Once Lois had undergone a thorough diagnostic evaluation, I broke the news to her and Saul that she had rapidly progressive Alzheimer's, with mild memory, language, and life skill loss. We then began the discussion about whether or not to tell family and friends. Lois believed that no one had noticed anything, unaware that it was her daughter Carrie's actions that had resulted in her visit to me. Neither she nor Saul wanted to share the diagnosis with anyone, including Carrie.

The MRI of Lois's brain revealed that she had had a few small strokes, likely over the preceding several years, although there was no way of knowing when they had occurred. Lois had no idea that she'd had them, which is not uncommon, as these so-called "silent strokes" can occur without any symptoms. However, they did not explain her cognitive condition, as they were too small and too few. Nonetheless, the three of us decided together that if people asked why Lois was forgetful, they would say it was from "mini-strokes." In my experience, people tend to react to a diagnosis of "strokes" much better than they do to a diagnosis of "Alzheimer's." A diagnosis of strokes is publicly perceived as more benign, although this is not always accurate. (Sometimes, even after I have given a patient a diagnosis of a type of dementia with a far worse prognosis than Alzheimer's, relieved patients and family members exclaim, "Thank God it's not Alzheimer's!")

Both Saul and Lois were adamant about not sharing the diagnosis with their family, despite being close to them. Knowing the backstory from Carrie, I asked, "Are you sure you don't want to tell your children?"

"No, we don't want to worry them," Saul said. This is a phrase that I hear often from patients and caregivers.

When Carrie called to inquire about her mother, I said, "Carrie, your parents do not want me to discuss the situation with anyone, including their children."

To her credit, Carrie pressed me no further, gleaning from my unsaid words what she wanted to know — that her mother was being treated for whatever it was that she had. In situations like these, my primary concern is the patient's right to confidentiality, but I am sensitive to the worries of loved ones.

Fast-forward a year, during which Lois, by the sheer force of her nature, had managed to keep up with a busy schedule summering on Cape Cod, wintering in Florida, and juggling her family's schedule in New York City in between. The entire time, Lois was confident that no one realized she had a problem. And outside of her immediate family and friends with whom she was in constant contact, that was probably true.

Around this time, however, I got a call another call from Carrie.

"I don't know what to do about Mom," she said. "She sat next to my son at his bar mitzvah, and that night he asked, 'Mom, does Grandma have Alzheimer's disease?' because he noticed that she kept repeating herself." Carrie added, "I think it's time for my mom to tell people she has Alzheimer's." She did not ask me if her mother did indeed have Alzheimer's disease — she already knew.

"I've come to know your mother," I responded, "and I feel that if she tells other people, it might break her spirit. What she has to go on now is her pride, and we've got to support her in that. She doesn't want to be labeled or defined by an illness; she wants people to see her as herself." In this

130

way, I was able to provide Carrie needed advice, without betraying Lois's trust.

Fortunately, I had more success in explaining this concept to Carrie than I'd had with Harold. She grasped my point immediately.

"You're right," Carrie said. "That would be a cruel thing to do to my mom. But can you please check with Mom and Dad again?"

I promised I would, and revisited the situation with Saul and Lois.

"Nobody has a clue," Saul said. "We have this thing covered. Everything is fine. No one knows, and we really don't think it's necessary to tell anyone."

Lois agreed. "If I thought that anybody knew, I would shut myself in the house and never go out again," she admitted.

I said that was fine, and we left it at that.

PEOPLE FIRST, PATIENTS SECOND
One reason I counsel patients to think twice before sharing a diagnosis of Alzheimer's is that the illness spectrum is still being discovered. We know that all strokes are not equal — that some strokes kill, others paralyze, and others merely inconvenience. But the common perception of Alzheimer's is shaped by the severe, advanced cases.

Both as physicians and as laypeople, we simply do not have the kind of knowledge about Alzheimer's that we do about some other well-known neurological conditions, like strokes or headaches.

Consider the fact that a hundred years ago, cervical cancer was the biggest killer of women. Now when women have cervical cancer, it's rarely a death sentence, and it certainly isn't perceived as such. Today we understand that there are gradations to this condition. We can also learn from the HIV and AIDS epidemic. When I was in training in the 1980s, being HIV positive was a death sentence. Now, three decades later, patients with HIV and AIDS are living full lives, even though there is still no cure. However, nuanced approaches to patients with Alzheimer's are not yet the norm. When people hear the word *Alzheimer's,* they conjure images of the most severe cases — people in nursing homes who can't speak and don't recognize their children.

The fact is that the majority of people with Alzheimer's disease are living functional lives in their communities. They may yet be on the mild end of the Alzheimer's spectrum. Or they may be obviously forgetful but still functioning members of society. They visit their new grandson from Kansas

City — a little absent-minded, perhaps, but perfectly able to bring home some ice cream from the local deli. They are repetitive at the bar mitzvah, but run three homes in three cities and coordinate a busy social schedule. They might forget appointments and what they had for breakfast, but remember the provenance of the earrings they're wearing.

Lois and Miriam deserve to be treated as unique people first, and patients second. Their Alzheimer's may progress to a point where it's clearly discernible to most people, and they may be forced to acknowledge it publicly, but they are still human beings with much to contribute and deserving of respect.

A few years ago, I went to an annual spring celebration for a large international marketing firm. The founder of the firm got up to give the speech, and the room full of savvy advertising professionals gave him their rapt attention. Everyone deified him. Although I happened to know that he had Alzheimer's (I was there at the behest of his wife, who was terrified that he was going to make a fool of himself), no one else in the room knew. I was not at all worried — in fact, I felt so confident that my patient could pull it off that I had actively encouraged him to do it. He had given hundreds, if not thousands, of speeches before, and I knew how much he wanted to give this one.

"If he wants to do this," I told his wife, "let him. It's his company and his hoorah."

My patient went up to the stage and started to give his speech. It was a typical spring evening event — the women wearing bright spring clothing, the windows open to let in the crisp evening air — yet my patient began by saying how Christmas was a time for reflection and introspection. I could see people in the room look a little puzzled for a moment, until they decided that he was probably getting at a larger message and was speaking metaphorically or in parables.

His wife and I were the only ones who knew that he was confused — that he thought it was the firm's annual Christmas celebration, not the spring gala. The rest of his speech went off without a hitch.

Afterward, people told him and his wife that it was one of the best speeches they'd ever heard, full of food for thought and wise aphorisms. But if the audience had known that he had Alzheimer's, the power of his words would have been lost. His initial mix-up would have colored the whole presentation. Because they didn't know, they saw him as they used to — as the founder of the company, a great communicator, a man who inspired and motivated them — and appreciated his wisdom. He was still able to move a room full of savvy marketing folk, despite his illness. It was an important illustration of why it's often best not to let people know.

SALLY TOLD EVERYONE!

Of course, there are exceptions to every rule. Sometimes with the not-telling comes a kind of fear, a fear of being "found out," the kind that gnawed at Lois and ate away at Harold's peace. To avoid this, some patients have opted to go with the "tell everyone" route, and have not suffered for doing so.

Sally, for example, smashed my advice to be circumspect about the diagnosis to smithereens. She was a vibrant 72-year-old with very white teeth, very pink lipstick, and very red hair. An actress and a natural-born charmer, she swept into my office with a dramatic flourish and a smile that had dazzled the waiting room.

Sally had been given a diagnosis of Alzheimer's disease by another doctor, but wanted a second opinion. I reviewed the notes from the thorough evaluation that she had already undergone with the other physician, a renowned specialist in the field.

"Sally," I said, "you went to an excellent doctor and he did all the right tests. I have to concur with his conclusion that you have Alzheimer's disease." I explained that I thought it was the slowly progressive kind, with mild memory loss and intact language and life skills.

"Well, all right, then — if I have it, I have it," Sally said with a briskness that I would come to love. "Let's get on with this business. Can anything be done about it?"

We discussed treatment options, and she took it all in stride.

Finally, I launched into my usual advice about not telling. "You have a very active and busy social life, Sally, and I should let you know that my approach is this: Keep this diagnosis to yourself."

I advised her that if anybody asked her about it, to be circumspect and to not mention Alzheimer's. I also told her to not bring up the issue of forgetfulness of her own accord either, because in my experience, the more someone says, "I'm forgetful," the more other people will notice it when it happens.

Sally agreed wholeheartedly, smiling happily. "Well, that makes perfect sense! It's no one's business but my own!"

A month later, Sally came back even more exuberant than she'd been when she had left me the first time.

"I've told everyone!" she declared. "My hairdresser knows. I've told my whole family . . . I even told my doormen." She flashed a triumphant smile. "You can't believe it! It has been a great experience."

I was horrified. "What?!" I sputtered. "You told *everyone*?"

She laughed. "Why, yes, darling, of course I did! What did you expect me to do?"

I realized then that she had forgotten our entire discussion about not telling others, remembering only the confirmation of her diagnosis.

"I make a joke of it," Sally continued. "Whenever I forget and someone says, 'What's the matter with you?' I say, 'What do you mean, what's the matter with me? I have Alzheimer's disease; that's what's the matter with me! Ha ha ha!' It's been great! You wouldn't believe the look on their faces — it shuts them right up. I forgot a theater appointment the other day, and my friend Teresa called me up, pissed to no end. I said to her, 'Teri, I have Alzheimer's!' Well, she ended up apologizing to me. I told her not to worry about it. And some people don't even believe I have Alzheimer's! One of my doormen said the other day, 'Sally, if you have Alzheimer's, I must have Alzheimer's too.' "

I think the reason this approach worked so well for Sally was that the way she delivered the news made people feel comfortable. It made them think: *Okay, maybe she does have this illness, but she's Sally first.* In that way, she's educating people, performing the important task of letting them know what the face of someone with Alzheimer's looks like. The next time Sally's friend Teresa or Sally's doorman meets someone who has Alzheimer's disease, the vision of someone staring blankly off into space will be supplanted by the image of a smiling, vibrant Sally. Sally's friend and her doormen will begin to grasp that Alzheimer's is a spectrum illness and that the existing stereotypes are far from the whole story.

ALZHEIMER'S IN THE COMMUNITY

I've demonstrated how people's perceptions of Alzheimer's can color their interaction with people with dementia — and not for the better. But Gina's story is an example of how communities can rise to the occasion and deliver walloping doses of kindness. Gina was 70 and overweight, with short black hair streaked with gray. She had rapidly progressive Alzheimer's disease, with mild memory loss and moderate-severe language and life skills impairment. On one of her visits to my office, she was wearing a neatly ironed red blouse, hanging loosely over black pants. Her eyes were brown and sparkly, although lately the sparkle came from the shimmer of unwept tears, stemming from anxiety and fear.

She wore brown eyeliner, blue eye shadow, and plum-colored lipstick and blush, all of which had been painstakingly applied by her husband, Joe, a retired cop. Joe was dressed in a navy blue suit with a crisp white shirt and geometric tie, his balding head shiny and his blue eyes resting on Gina as often as they rested on me. His large abdomen was barely restrained by his suit jacket.

"I told her I was putting her in one of those nursing homes if she don't start behaving," Joe said.

Gina looked wordlessly at Joe, shook her head, and then turned to me, her lips trembling, "I don't . . . don't . . . ."

"Gina," I said, "if he keeps teasing you like that, I would give him a good punch."

"Y-ye-yeah," Gina said, smiling. When she smiled, her whole face became luminous, her eyes crinkling at the corners.

We were sitting in my office. I was behind my desk, and Joe and Gina were across from me, beside each other.

"We're late because of her," Joe said, jerking his head toward Gina. Joe hated being late. They were generally at my office a good half hour before the scheduled appointment time.

"She got up before she was done on the toilet this morning," he went on. "I know she was trying to help me out, Doc, but Doc, it was all over the place — the floors, her clothes, everything. You know what I'm saying — the stuff was everywhere. She was already dressed, and I had to put her back in the shower and clean her up . . . clean the place up . . . clean myself up. And yeah, I yelled at her. I yelled and I screamed . . . I'm not saying I didn't . . . I know she don't mean it, but I couldn't help myself."

Gina's eyes were beginning to shimmer, and Joe, although he was looking at and talking to me, reached for her hand and held it.

"I . . . yeah, I . . . I . . ." Gina stuttered.

"Yes, Gina?" I said encouragingly as she tried to speak despite her difficulties, but Joe interrupted.

"My daughter came up from downstairs, hollering at me," Joe went on. "Told me I

140

was a horrible man . . . I told her 'Shut up! If you care so much about your mother, why don't you help out more?' "

Joe and Gina's adult daughter lived in the basement of their single-family home in Long Island and, busy with her own life, spent very little time with them. Gina shook her head as Joe said this.

"My worry is that if this happened at work, that won't be no good," Joe said. "It may be the end of the road. I may have to stop bringing her in."

Gina's eyes widened, and she started shaking her head. Joe took Gina to work with him every day in Brooklyn in his postretirement job as head of security for a large not-for-profit group. Gina had initially volunteered there, stuffing envelopes and fetching coffee for the staff. Now she simply walked the long corridors, smiling at everyone.

"They all love her at work, they would do anything for Gina, but this . . . this . . . They may say I can't bring her in no more, and I can't say I would do any different in their shoes."

Gina began to fidget in her chair, almost rocking.

"You may have to find another solution," I said. "Gina, this may not be as bad as you think. We can get someone to stay at home with you."

Gina looked at me in alarm, her face twisted, shaking her head. She started crying. "No . . . no . . . no . . . like . . . nice . . . Joe . . ."

Joe turned completely toward Gina and gazed at her for a long minute. High school sweethearts, they had been married for decades. "For better or worse, like we promised back then . . . She'll always be my girl," Joe was fond of repeating. "Yeah, you drive me nuts, Gina, you know." He squeezed her hand and turned back toward me. "She really likes coming to work with me, Doc, and the people there, they haven't said anything so far . . ." His voice trailed off.

I saw how they were seated together, facing me, having moved their chairs to within inches of each other. I saw how he struggled to understand this strange new world that she now inhabited and to make sense of the topsy-turvy world that he found himself in. I saw how Gina tried to make herself heard and how she tried so hard to be "good." I saw the helpless distress each felt in causing grief in the other. I felt the strength in their gaze.

"Gina," I said finally. "We will figure it

out. You keep on going to work with Joe like you want. We will deal with whatever comes up."

Gina started laughing through her tears. "I love you!" she said to me. It was her only complete sentence during that visit.

Later that year, I went to Joe and Gina's fiftieth wedding anniversary celebration. It was at an Italian restaurant filled with people who loved them both and understood Gina's condition. Gina stood beside Joe and greeted everyone with a smile. She was having a grand time. When it was time to eat, we had to cut the food for her, but no one cared. It was community at its best. And that community support spilled over into their daily lives. The restaurants that Joe and Gina frequented knew of her diagnosis and made sure to seat them in a quiet place. Her longtime manicurist was especially gentle with Gina and even came to visit her at home once in a while so Joe could take a break. Joe's coworkers were friendly and kind to Gina and found chores for her — stacking papers, putting away provisions — so she would feel needed. Everyone knew that Gina had Alzheimer's disease, and the limitations it imposed on her were plain to see, but people could also see the happiness in Gina's face and the love between Joe and Gina.

"I like being with her," said Gina's manicurist, whom I met at the dinner. "I can totally be myself. I know it sounds crazy but it's true. I don't have to pretend about anything. If I'm sad, she's sad with me. When I'm happy, she laughs. I really enjoy her company."

It's my hope that as time goes on and more is revealed about Alzheimer's, public perception of the disease will change. This is especially important because dementia affects so many of us. Like the general population, if I live into my mideighties, I will have a more than 50 percent chance of developing Alzheimer's. My odds of developing the disease would be more about "when" than "if." I wouldn't want those who are aware of my diagnosis to start treating me like I'm an idiot, to talk around me when I'm with them and incorrectly assume I'm not capable of grasping things. I want them to understand that Alzheimer's has many faces and that no matter how the condition manifests in patients, we are all deserving of respect.

I'm optimistic that in thirty years' time, the fear and stigma surrounding Alzheimer's will be a thing of the past and there will be increasingly effective treatments.

If and when I am told that I have Alzheimer's, I pray I will have the self-confidence of Sally and Miriam, the support of a partner like Saul, and the love of a community as accepting and supportive as Gina's.

CHAPTER 4
DO I NEED TO QUIT MY JOB? CONTINUING TO WORK WITH DEMENTIA — AND KNOWING WHEN TO RETIRE

"Can I keep working?" This tends to be one of the first things newly diagnosed Alzheimer's patients ask me. Concerns about their performance at work are often what prompted their initial visit, and they're eager to know whether they'll be able to continue to earn a living and practice their trade.

Whenever possible, I answer yes.

It is important to understand that a dementia diagnosis does not automatically disqualify a person from working. Depending on what type of dementia a person has and what skills are affected, he or she may be able to continue to work for many years. The first step is to determine which cognitive areas are affected by the dementia (this varies with the type of dementia and where on the spectrum the patient falls) and compare that with the skills required by the particular job. What kind of job is it? How long has the person performed it? Is the job hands-on or is it supervisory? Does it require a skill set that the patient has retained, based on their neurocognitive evaluation? What would the consequenses be if the patient made a mistake? What support systems does the patient have in place? For example, is there an assistant who can remind them about meetings and function as an ancillary memory system? These and numerous other variables are analyzed in making decisions about continuing to work.

When I see a person with Alzheimer's disease, I start by asking myself whether I would trust his or her judgment. Where on the Alzheimer's spectrum do they fall? Would I take myself or my family to see them in their profession? I base my assessment on an evaluation of their judgment after a thorough neurologic, neurocognitive, and laboratory examination, with close follow-up to monitor disease progression.

If someone is very skilled in their job and has been at it a long time, their work becomes an "over-learned" memory, which means that it is stored in multiple areas of the brain and is usually affected much later in the course of Alzheimer's. Practice makes perfect, and the longer we do something, the more skilled we become at it. Such long-term work skills function similarly to the generally preserved skills of being able to eat, walk, and drive.

To demonstrate the process I use to make a determination of a patient's ability to keep working, I will start off by discussing physicians with dementia. This is because in my role as a consultant to the New York State Committee on Physician Health, I have had a chance to delve deeply into this question. Additionally, the thought of someone with Alzheimer's practicing medicine is particularly jarring to many of us. *How could I ever entrust my health to someone with dementia?* we might ask ourselves. After that, I will discuss patients in some other professions. Also, keep in mind the patients mentioned in earlier chapters — Joe, the money manager; Bella, the pension fund manager; and Megan, the administrative head of a private firm — who are all thriving in their jobs despite a diagnosis of Alzheimer's.

A PSYCHIATRIST WITH ALZHEIMER'S

Dr. Samuels was an 82-year-old psychiatrist who maintained his professional skills even as his memory loss progressed. Despite his dementia he had a full roster of patients. His wife was incredulous.

"*Who* are these *idiots* still paying to see my husband?" Doris exclaimed during one of our conversations. "He can't even take a telephone message for me, for crying out loud. He forgets from one minute to the next. How can these people, who are supposed to be so smart, still come to see him? He answers the door in his pajamas, for God's sake!"

Dr. Samuels was a world-renowned analyst — he had the ability to talk to a patient for twenty to twenty-five minutes and immediately identify some of the major issues that person was struggling with. His interpretive skills were so superb that I sometimes asked him questions about my own practice. His advice was always on target.

The doctor had an impressive roster of discerning patients, men and women who were pillars of New York's business world and at the peak of their professional lives. He prided himself on his ability to coach them through difficult transactions at work and home.

Dr. Samuels saw his patients at his home office, and unfortunately, as his Alzheimer's progressed, he began to forget that he had made appointments. Time and again, these accomplished businessmen and businesswomen would ring his doorbell and he would answer in his bathrobe.

Interestingly, the doctor's professional

demeanor was such that his patients thought nothing of such lapses. They would go into their session regardless of his attire and leave satisfied with the level of care they had received. His practice continued to thrive.

The reason was simple: Dr. Samuels was still an exceptional analyst. He had spent his whole life making interpretations, and he was still good at it. Even if he wasn't able to keep an appointment book, take down phone messages, or remember to change into professional clothes, he maintained the skills necessary to help his patients.

Dr. Samuels, who sought me out when he realized that his memory was failing, was not surprised to hear that he had slowly progressive Alzheimer's, with mild-moderate memory loss and good language and life skills. "I suspected as much," he said.

Because his analytic skills were excellent, we agreed that he could continue to practice. We also agreed that he would give up prescribing medications. I felt that there was too much risk of prescription errors, given his memory loss, and Dr. Samuels concurred.

Dr. Samuels continued to practice in this manner for seven more years, finding meaning in his life and being of use to others until the ripe old age of 89, when he decided to retire.

Our episodic memories, ones that recall "where" and "when" — the memories with the shortest brain "shelf life" — are the most perishable for everyone, including for patients with Alzheimer's. I may remember a conversation I had with a friend, but it is harder for me to recall exactly when I had it. I may know that I'm supposed to meet a cousin for dinner, but not remember where to meet her.

Similarly, Dr. Samuels remembered that he was seeing patients, but forgot the "when" of it. Nonetheless, he retained his memories for over-learned facts and for procedures, which in his case was making the right analytic interpretations of various behaviors. This kind of knowledge is far more durable in all of us. We don't forget how to ride a bicycle, and neither do people with Alzheimer's. We may forget when we saw a beautiful rose and exactly where it was, but we know what a rose is — an over-learned fact — and so do most patients on the spectrum.

Less rehearsed facts, like the name of the capital of Morocco — or, in Dr. Samuels's case, the available dosages of Xanax — are

HOW THE BRAIN STORES MEMORY

This is a simplified schematic of the different types of memory, where they are stored in the brain, and how they are affected in aging and in Alzheimer's and other dementias.

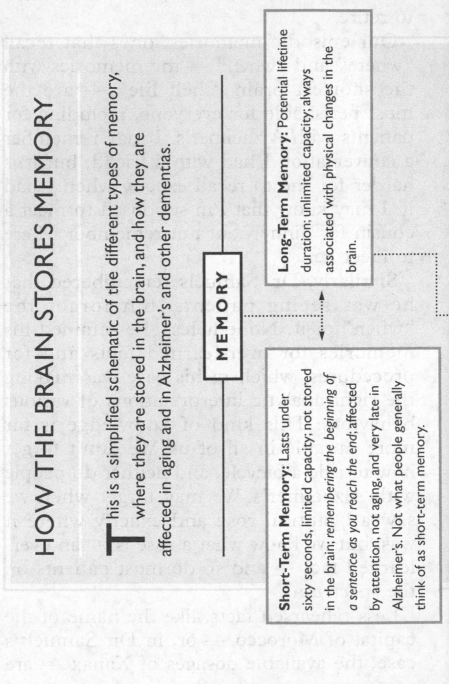

MEMORY

Short-Term Memory: Lasts under sixty seconds, limited capacity; not stored in the brain; *remembering the beginning of a sentence as you reach the end*; affected by attention, not aging, and very late in Alzheimer's. Not what people generally think of as short-term memory.

Long-Term Memory: Potential lifetime duration; unlimited capacity; always associated with physical changes in the brain.

Explicit (Declarative) Memory: Conscious "spoken" memory; needs specific brain processing areas to store new memories and to retrieve old ones; *the memory required to pass exams.*

Semantic (Factual) Memory: General facts; *What's a synonym for "good?" What is my date of birth? What is my sister's name?;* affected later in Alzheimer's, not by aging.

Implicit (Procedural) Memory: Unconscious "muscle" or "how" memory; stored throughout the brain; how to dance; how to play the piano; *how to navigate courtroom procedure for an experienced lawyer;* resistant to destruction; affected late in Alzheimer's and not by aging.

Episodic (Event) Memory: Associated with specific moments in time; *What's his name? Where and when did I speak with him last?* What people commonly—and inaccurately—call "short-term memory." Affected in many conditions including normal forgetting, aging, and early in Alzheimer's.

153

harder to retain for people both with and without memory impairment. Dr. Samuels's episodic memory for remembering appointments was almost nonexistent. But he recognized his patients and remembered their stories. His psychoanalytical skills and his memory of the ins and outs of different psychiatric interventions and procedures were still superb, and that was what his patients needed from him.

A Devoted Doctor

Dr. Bailey is a magnificent example of what patients on the spectrum are capable of. She was in her late thirties by the time she qualified as a doctor, having had two earlier careers as a teacher and a nurse. Practicing medicine was her life goal, so of course, Dr. Bailey was thrilled when she finally achieved her ambition. Her dedication to her practice was evident in the close relationships and bonds she maintained with her patients.

As Dr. Bailey got older, she spent less time seeing patients at her office and more time teaching academic medicine in a university hospital, but caring for the patients she did see still meant the world to her. As her practice became smaller, she ended up functioning as an almost private physician for some very complex patients with chronic conditions, including post-traumatic stress disorder and psychological issues resulting from a history of sexual abuse. These long-term patients relied on Dr. Bailey and trusted her with their lives. In turn, she was fiercely dedicated to them.

By the age of 75, though, Dr. Bailey was having trouble with her memory. A social worker with whom she worked and whom she'd known since her nursing days advised Dr. Bailey to seek help. She went to a memory disorders center at another hospital in the region. She was diagnosed with Alzheimer's and was told she would have to give up her practice right away. She was absolutely devastated.

By the time of our first meeting, Dr. Bailey was beyond depressed. She hadn't had a chance to say goodbye to her patients, and she was worried that some, particularly those with major trust issues given their difficult pasts, were not being given enough time to find another physician.

Dr. Bailey decided to seek assistance from the New York State Committee on Physician Health, which is how we came to meet. This committee was formed to evaluate medical professionals who are suspected of having health issues that interfere with their ability to practice. Instead of being punitive, the committee seeks to assist referred physicians by getting them the right treatment and when possible helping them return to their jobs. Usually hospital administrators ask for an evaluation, often as a result of departmental staff expressing concern about the physician's judgment. In some rare cases the affected physicians themselves request the evaluation. I am part of the group of consultants that assesses such patients on behalf of the committee.

When Dr. Bailey came to see me, she had already given up her teaching responsibilities, which I was privately upset about. I could tell she had been a wonderful teacher, and giving up the medical practice made more sense to me than giving up teaching. However, I quickly came to understand that the doctor felt a greater obligation to her patients than her students. She was too invested in her patients to just cut them loose without a firm follow-up plan in place.

Once I tested Dr. Bailey, I realized that she was still remarkably intelligent — she scored at the 98th percentile overall in terms of her cognitive ability, compared with healthy women of her age. She also had enough memory and cognitive wherewithal to function at a reasonable and safe level. I told her that, with supervision, she could continue practicing as long as her charts were reviewed every month by another physician, and on the grounds that she not take on any new patients. She was so happy and relieved that she burst into tears right there in my office.

"You have no idea how wonderful it is to be listened to," she said softly. "I have tried to be that kind of doctor myself. You heard my concerns. Thank you."

I felt myself getting teary too. Heartfelt compliments from physician patients are the hardest to come by, and the ones I prize the most.

Dr. Bailey continued to work and take care of her patients for three more years, under close supervision of another physician. Over the course of the last year of her practice, Dr. Bailey broke the news of her Alzheimer's to her patients and succeeded in placing each of them with another physician she knew they would get along with.

During this process, she told me, "This feels right. I'm glad I can take care of them in the way that they trusted me to." And right before she finally retired, she said, "You know, I think I'm ready to say goodbye to medicine."

I remember feeling good about this unexpected statement. As did Dr. Bailey. It was time for her to say goodbye to something she had given so much of her life to, and she was able to do so with grace, honoring her relationship with her beloved patients.

After she left her practice, Dr. Bailey didn't slow down much. She started writing a memoir, which kept her busy and allowed her a dignified exit from a practice in which she remained capable up to the very end. In Dr. Bailey's case, not only was there no reason for an abrupt departure, but to force one on her would've been a disaster for both her and her patients.

In a funny twist to the story that speaks to how many patients on the spectrum continue to work and work well, Dr. Bailey's own physician, with whom I had conferred extensively during her illness, turned out to have Alzheimer's as well, and retired from his practice about six months before his death. Neither Dr. Bailey nor I had had any inkling that he was having problems. Sometimes, he took a little longer to return my calls, and on occasion I had to reiterate things to him, but I recalled this only in hindsight. At the time, I had no clue that there was anything wrong with him, and he took good care of Dr. Bailey until his retirement.

A SURGEON WITH ALZHEIMER'S

Whereas Dr. Bailey's story ended well, Dr. Alan's did not. He was a 63-year-old orthopedic surgeon who had called himself "a knee man" for the majority of his career. He examined knees, he injected knees, he repaired knees, he replaced knees. Knees were Dr. Alan's professional life.

"Knees are a puzzle in the joint world," he said. "They take a real beating and are structurally the most flimsily put together of the joints."

When he began to have trouble remembering, the first person to notice was his transcriptionist. Dr. Alan's handwriting had been notoriously bad his whole life, so he had an on-site transcriptionist who took notes while he saw patients. The transcriptionist noticed that Dr. Alan sometimes asked patients the same question several times and on occasion forgot aspects of a just-told history. She mentioned it to the office manager, and shortly thereafter, Dr. Alan saw a memory disorders specialist and was diagnosed with Alzheimer's.

He was then referred to me by a friend for another opinion. After a thorough evaluation that included a neurocognitive assessment, I agreed with the original diagnosis. When Dr. Alan and his wife, Emily, arrived to hear the results, I informed them that he had slowly progressive Alzheimer's disease, with mild-moderate memory loss and good language and life skills.

One of Emily's first questions was "How long can he keep working?"

Dr. Alan himself was reticent, and it appeared that in their relationship, his wife was the one who spoke on their behalf and made decisions for the couple.

When asked directly, Dr. Alan concurred that he was curious about how long he could keep working.

"I don't think you can continue much longer, because your memory issues are already impacting your work," I replied.

Unlike Dr. Samuels, who knew his psycho-analytic patients well and agreed to stop prescribing, and unlike Dr. Bailey with her small group of long-term patients and her excellent overall function, Dr. Alan had a busy practice with new patients showing up daily. Furthermore, on his cognitive evaluation, his memory was at the 10th percentile and his overall ability was at the 30th percentile compared with other healthy men in his age group. His was also a higher-risk practice, as he had to make diagnoses, prescribe medications, and perform procedures on patients he had just met.

Emily again characteristically responded on behalf of her husband: "But he doesn't even do very much surgery. Most of his procedures are routine."

I explained to her that she was right in that most of those procedures were like "muscle" or "procedural" memories for Dr. Alan, so they were actually much more resistant to deterioration by Alzheimer's disease. He had done so many knee replacements that he could likely do them by rote. I did, however, remain concerned that he may not be able to provide the best care for his patients given his cognitive status.

At my insistence, his wife reluctantly agreed to have her husband stop operating. I decided that his in-office procedures were so familiar and automatic to him, thanks to his life as a "knee man," that Dr. Alan was capable of continuing those.

In an effort to prolong her husband's working life, Emily pitched in around the office, as did all Dr. Alan's staff members. Emily attempted to compensate for Dr. Alan's memory issues by double-checking the transcriptionist's notes and making sure the prescriptions were correct. She became a de facto second office manager. However, Emily had no medical training, and the strain of her constant double-checking was hard on their marriage. The impulse on the part of family members and coworkers to jump in and help — to try to function as ancillary memory systems or overseers — is understandable. It arises from that most human of tendencies: to help someone in need. In this case, though, I was not sure that the effort was worth the outcome.

The three of us discussed various options for treatment. What struck me was that, despite Emily's eagerness to have her husband continue working, she showed a clear lack of enthusiasm for him getting any extra treatment if it was going to incur financial costs in lost patient time. So Dr. Alan went without enrolling in any of the newer trials and didn't try any of the off-label treatments, such as TMS or cognitive exercises. Despite my suggestions, Dr. Alan received only the standard available medications, donepezil and memantine. I suspected that Emily was leery of clinical trials because she was worried that the time commitment required would interfere with his continued working.

Dr. Alan's memory loss continued to be a problem, and within six months it was apparent that it was not safe for him to continue to practice. He sent out letters to his patients announcing his retirement.

Unfortunately, I do not know what happened to Dr. Alan, as he left my care after his retirement.

A LAWYER WITH ALZHEIMER'S

Ryan was a 64-year-old attorney with his own small but flourishing legal firm that focused on wills and real-estate law. He was married and lived with his wife and three of his five children, who ranged in age from 12 to 25.

He came to see me because he had been having trouble retrieving words and was finding himself forgetful during meetings. His difficulties were becoming apparent to some of his clients. Ryan had been able to compensate for it, thanks to his two paralegals and a partner, all of whom had worked with him for many years and were devoted to him. They picked up the slack as Ryan's condition got worse, as Dr. Alan's staff had done with him. However, despite their efforts, it did finally reach a point where Ryan knew he needed medical assistance.

I diagnosed Ryan with rapidly progressive Alzheimer's with mild language and memory difficulties and good life skills.

"What am I going to do?" he said, his eyes filling with tears. "My wife and I haven't saved enough for me to retire. Besides, my youngest is only 12, and I'm still paying for college for two of my other children. I have to keep working."

I put Ryan on an aggressive treatment protocol. In addition to medication, we started him on off-label treatment with TMS. However, when he underwent repeat testing in six months to assess response to treatment, it was clear that his memory had deteriorated. Treatment had unfortunately failed to stem the progression of Ryan's Alzheimer's.

In his last year at the practice, Ryan was open about his condition to his clients as Dr. Bailey had been with her patients toward the end of her tenure.

"I have Alzheimer's," he would say, maintaining an authoritative air. "You must help me if I forget."

Help him they did, until it was no longer possible for him to practice safely. Ryan retired about two years after his diagnosis and he has needed increasingly more help at home as his cognition has continued to deteriorate.

When Telling at Work Backfires
Sometimes, of course, elements of our support systems may fail us, as in the case of Ellie, a tenured college professor of educa-

tion. She was 58 but she looked much younger because of her slight figure, hopeful eyes, and her hair, which she wore tied back in a ponytail. She came from a small, working-class family in Queens, and was the first person in her family to have graduated from college. Not only that, but she went on to get her doctorate and teach at a prestigious university.

Ellie came to see me at the behest of her psychiatrist. She had sought psychiatric help for the recent onset of a vague anxiety and depression, the cause of which she could not put her finger on. Her psychiatrist treated her for depression, but Ellie continued to have trouble managing her course schedule, even though she had been teaching the same courses for twenty years. The psychiatrist became concerned that this was something more than depression and referred her to me.

When I saw Ellie, I felt like I wanted to protect her. There was something endearing, vulnerable, and almost childlike about her. After testing, I discovered that she had rapidly progressive Alzheimer's with mild language and memory loss and good life skills.

Ellie was still teaching a full course load at her school. Even though she had been experiencing some difficulty, she'd actually been given extra classes to teach in the upcoming semester. After discussing her diagnosis, I advised Ellie not to tell anyone at work about her condition.

"Do you like your job?" I asked.

"I love it."

"Well, then, be circumspect. I suggest you think very carefully about whom you tell. People who don't understand that Alzheimer's is a spectrum disorder might think that you aren't competent to teach anymore."

The next time I saw Ellie, she had a big smile on her face.

"You know, Dr. Devi, I am so relieved," she said, ponytail bobbing.

"What do you mean?"

"Well, after I left your office last time, I felt I was not being true to the people at my job by not telling them. So, at our staff meeting, I announced that the reason I had been so quiet for the last year was that I had Alzheimer's. I would rather they know than think me stupid. They couldn't have been more supportive. I went to see my supervisor. She is usually a very cold woman. But when I told her I had Alzheimer's, she came around from behind her desk and gave me a big hug. I felt so understood."

"Ellie, I'm so happy for you," I said. "I'm very glad that I was wrong. I am delighted that a big university system can be so nurturing."

Unfortunately, the story did not end there. A month later, when I next saw Ellie, she told me that her supervisor had called her into her office, where several of her colleagues were waiting. They told her they had reviewed the student evaluations from the previous two years. Based on those evaluations, they had decided that she could no longer continue teaching.

Even though they had been giving Ellie extra courses to teach before she shared her diagnosis with them, once they were informed, they began to look at her through what I call "Alzheimer's-colored lenses" and told her almost immediately that she must go on disability. Ellie's is a sad story, but it illustrates how important it is to figure out whom to tell and when to tell them, particularly in the workplace.

A Professor Who Made Words Dance

My patient, Professor Mather, was a tenured university lecturer who had written many textbooks on the subject of etymology and lived with slowly progressive Alzheimer's for sixteen years. Shortly before his death at 88, he couldn't tell me what time of the day it was or what month or year it was, but he still was able to give me the definition of *polemical.* In fact, his vocabulary as a patient with Alzheimer's far surpassed that of most people without dementia. He had retired from active teaching in his late fifties, and focused instead on writing textbooks, which he did well because of his retained language skills and his over-learned knowledge of his field.

Because of the human tendency to "box and label," we may dismiss the entirety of a person's intellect based on an area of deficit, a type of negative halo effect. With Professor Mather, for example, one might have dismissed his overall intellect simply because of his poor memory — he would do things like forget and ask for dessert just after his dessert plate had been cleared. But if one accepted that Professor Mather's memory for recent events and time was poor, and focused instead on other aspects such as his prodigious intelligence, spirited and enlightening discussions invariably resulted. If the negative halo effect was done away with, a listener could get engrossed in a history of exactly how the word *escape* was derived from the Latin *ex* "out" and *cappa* "cloak," or about dybbuks, malicious spirits of the dead.

My point is that even sixteen years into his diagnosis, I would have welcomed Professor Mather as my English professor. Over the many years I saw him, we would engage in wordplay for a few minutes toward the end of his visits. This appealed to both of us. It made him feel more competent and less like a patient, and it made me feel less like his doctor and more like his student. In those exchanges, we broke out of our prescribed roles and became individuals to each other.

Professor Mather made words and their etymological roots dance before my eyes, tweaking them here and there, a master puppeteer like no other. I watched words dissolve and reconsolidate as entirely new apparitions, new shoots from the same roots. The magic he wove with words was sublime, and to this day, I remember the words he taught me. Before I knew him, I had never used an etymological dictionary; now I always do when I need to look up a word. Despite having Alzheimer's, he made my vocabulary stronger and enriched my life.

WHICH JOB FOR WHICH PATIENT?

Because Alzheimer's is a spectrum disorder that causes a multitude of symptoms as varied as the functions of the brain, its presentation varies significantly from individual to individual. As a result, the ability to function at a job depends on the symptoms a patient has. You can have a maestro fully able to teach a master class despite not remembering the names of his grandchildren. You can have a doorman who remembers his family but no longer has a memory for faces, and thus is having trouble at work. If the doorman had mild difficulties with word retrieval without loss of facial recognition, however, he could continue to function, meeting and greeting building dwellers and their guests.

We must learn to assess a patient's ability to continue to work by evaluating the symptoms of the particular individual and how those symptoms pertain to the requirements of their job. As I mentioned earlier, someone who has spent years becoming highly skilled at their job, whether it be carpentry or neurosurgery, incorporates and weaves this skill into the very fabric of their brain, literally hardwiring it, forming procedural memories that are resistant to destruction from disease processes. This is how

Professor Mather retained his knowledge of complex words and Dr. Samuels retained his analytic skills.

You may also remember Bella, my pension fund manager. She developed Alzheimer's at age 75, and five years later she was still managing my pension plan with admirable results. Her ability to balance funds was over-learned and was now procedural, as automatic to Bella as diagnosing neurologic illness is to me.

A PRESIDENT WITH DEMENTIA?

An example that I like to mention to patients is President Ronald Reagan. At age 22 Reagan was hired for his first job as a radio announcer because his memory was so phenomenal. He was able to give a play-by-play account of an entire football game from memory.

But his memory had discernibly begun to fail toward the end of his first term as president. Running for reelection, he had difficulty with words and fumbled during televised debates. Although Reagan was diagnosed only in 1994 with Alzheimer's, five years after he left office, recent research revealed that during his first and second terms he had word-finding difficulties that are often seen early in the course of Alzheimer's.

During one memorable televised debate, Reagan appeared visibly confused. By the time of the Iran–Contra hearings in 1985–87, the once exceptionally articulate president took to the stand to say over and over again that he could not remember. Some viewed this as the standard defense of a seasoned politician on trial, but the president may have been telling the truth. His son, Ron Reagan, asserted that his father had Alzheimer's as early as 1984, though this claim has been refuted by the president's doctors.

Having watched tapes of President Reagan's public speeches and noticed his increasing reliance on notes and vagueness in responses over time, it is my opinion that he may have been developing symptoms on the spectrum while still serving as president. Nonetheless, few in the American public had any inkling of an impending problem, despite the president's numerous televised appearances. It is important to note that in President Reagan's case, no diagnosis was made until he was several years out of office.

THRIVING WITH TREATMENT AND SUPPORT

Most people who develop Alzheimer's can live productive lives for many years into the illness, given the right medical treatment and support systems. Such systems include family, friends, and colleagues as well as neighbors and larger communities. Support can best be provided when we prevent the negative halo effect from clouding our perception and enjoy what the patient retains, rather than bemoaning what they have lost. This helps maintain the confidence of patients who feel vulnerable about potential intellectual compromise. Also, friends, family, and communities can serve as ancillary cognitive systems when required, for example by helping fill in memory gaps and providing missing words or smoothing over lapses. Professionals, including physicians like myself, can make a difference in the quality of life for the patient by prescribing treatment to stabilize the illness. Supporting the family caregiver and helping to prevent their burnout and depression is also essential.

The truth is, no matter how well we educate people about Alzheimer's or how much support a patient has, people may be leery about having someone with dementia continue to work. Would you let an accountant with Alzheimer's file your taxes? Would you be willing to have someone with Alzheimer's drive your daughter's school bus? Would you let your mechanic with dementia work on your car? For that matter, what about your mechanic who had a stroke or a brain tumor? Or your mechanic who is receiving chemotherapy or has epilepsy or suffers from substance abuse problems? My guess is that many of us may say yes to many conditions, but no to dementia, which is perceived to pose greater cognitive problems. Although that may be true in some patients on the Alzheimer's spectrum, it is not the case for the majority.

It's also worth noting that alongside an electrician with Alzheimer's whose judgment may be superb, there are many electricians whose judgment is questionable, even without any cognitive impairment. We all bring varied innate talents to each of our jobs, and we don't all start from a level playing field.

What I have learned about working with dementia is that a good evaluation can help determine the feasibility of continuing to work, perhaps with some extra support systems or work-arounds in place. Although enlightened organizations like the Committee on Physician Health are able to appreciate this reality, other organizations, such as the university where Ellie worked, are unable to do so. Once we grasp that Alzheimer's is a spectrum disorder, it is easier to allow for variability in the illness and support the patient in their wish to continue to work. Of course, as for all patients, careful monitoring over time is necessary.

As stated earlier, it can help to think about dementia in relation to conditions like epilepsy, bipolar disorder, or stroke, all of which may affect thinking and cognition. Because we understand the variability associated with those conditions, we allow many people suffering from them to continue to work and find value and purpose in their lives. It is my hope that we will soon be able to do this for people with Alzheimer's as well.

CHAPTER 5
WHO SAYS I CAN'T DRIVE?
MAINTAINING INDEPENDENCE
AND DIGNITY IN ALZHEIMER'S

"What do you mean I can't drive?" Ina exclaimed, furious. "That is the most ridiculous thing I've ever heard!"

She turned to her children for support. "Did you hear what she said? Tell her what a good driver I am! Tell her I have never had a single violation or ticket, ever!"

Ina was reacting to a perceived threat to her independence. Deciding how we spend our time, where we go, and whom we see are essential to feeling free and in control of our destiny. For many patients, loss of independence is one of the things they fear most. There are many ways to maintain independence in dementia, including living in your own home, choosing what to eat, and choosing how to spend your money. But I've found that one of the touchiest issues — the source of many heated arguments and tears in my office — is driving, as was the case with Ina.

What Ina said was true. She did have an impeccable driving record, far better than almost anyone I knew, including myself. At 86, she had been driving for sixty-seven years. In fact, she had insisted on driving her son and daughter into the city for her appointment from Long Island. Earlier in the visit, I'd told her about her Alzheimer's diagnosis. She received the news very calmly. She was composed as I told her about medications she would need to take, asking a couple of questions about the side effects but otherwise seeming at ease. When I told her she had to stop driving, however, Ina reacted as if I had driven a spear into her soul. She sprang forward like a cat and placed her hands on my desk to register her protest.

Her children had privately confessed to me over the phone before the visit that Ina seemed more hesitant on the road, less confident than usual. At the time I was just five years into my practice, and her family's concerns coupled with her diagnosis made it easy for me to determine that Ina should stop driving.

"Mom," her son said, placing his hand on her arm, "maybe this would be for the best. We can drive you where you need to go — it will give us a chance to spend more time with you."

"What are you talking about?" his mother said, snatching her arm away from him, sensing a conspiracy. "This is nonsense. I won't stop driving, and that is all we shall say about it." She glared at me. "And that goes for you too, Doctor!"

Ina didn't actually do all that much driving, even though she lived in suburban Long Island. The only places she drove to regularly were her synagogue and the supermarket — both quite close to her home. She went out three to four times a week, at most. Even so, Ina was utterly devastated.

Once she got home, she forgot nearly all the details of her visit with me except that she had, for some unclear reason, been told to stop driving, and this by a doctor she had seen just twice. The whole matter irritated and angered her. She appealed to her internist of twenty-odd years.

"They think that I shouldn't drive anymore," she told him. "You don't agree, do you?" He gently told her he thought it would be best if she stopped. Nonetheless, Ina continued to drive defiantly and, in her defense, carefully and without incident. Ina had been driving for so long that it was a procedural memory skill, deeply embedded in the neural circuits of her brain and relatively resistant to destruction by Alzheimer's pathology. Nonetheless, her family became increasingly worried about her continued driving, not because of any noticeable deterioration in her driving skills, but because of her diagnosis. They appealed to me again, and I came up with the idea of telling Ina that her car needed to be taken in for servicing. Each time Ina called the garage, the mechanics were instructed to come up with another excuse for why the car could not be used. This might seem manipulative and mean, but we — the family and myself — thought it would have been even more devastating to Ina to be forcibly stopped from driving. We felt it was less confrontational; this way she could blame her mechanics, but she saw through our tactics.

Each time she spoke to her son or daughter, she asked the same thing: "When am I getting my car back?"

Slowly but surely, Ina grew more depressed, more withdrawn, and more helpless. She stopped eating and lost interest in almost everything, and died within six months. To this day I firmly believe that I was partially responsible for her death. By colluding to keep her from driving, merely because she had received a dementia diagnosis, we had succeeded in taking away something crucial to Ina: her sense of independence.

Ina's case prompted me to do a lot of soul-searching, and she, like so many of my patients, proved to be an able teacher. I dived into the literature on driving and the elderly and on driving and dementia, and what I discovered not only surprised me, but changed my practice for the better.

The reality is that older drivers, including many patients on the Alzheimer's spectrum, are, for the most part, still more competent on the road than young people who have just obtained their license. Statistically, in fact, the group with the highest number of accidents and fatalities overall are drivers in their thirties. Older drivers are safer because they drive more slowly and for shorter distances, and well-publicized tragic exceptions aside, fatalities among elderly drivers generally do not involve other people. Because patients with Alzheimer's retain memory for procedures like driving, most can continue to drive safely until their illness progresses to the point that their reaction times and decision-making skills are impaired.

There are, of course, very clear-cut cases of patients with dementia who should not be driving. One such was my patient Dave. He was a 64-year-old carpenter who described himself to everyone he met as "ebullient and enthusiastic" before letting out a big, contagious laugh. Every time he arrived in my office, he high-fived everyone in the waiting room, much to their surprise. With my older, frailer patients, it sometimes seemed as if he might literally knock them down with his enthusiasm. He was quirky and insisted on being called by his first name. If I used his last name, which I was more comfortable with, he simply refused to answer.

After extensive testing, I determined that Dave had a type of frontotemporal dementia, which affects the brain's frontal lobes and interferes with judgment and social interactions more than with memory, particularly early in the disease process. This is the reverse of what is commonly seen in Alzheimer's. The pathology in frontotemporal dementia is also different, with few of the plaque deposits found in Alzheimer's. The earliest signs in Dave's case were that he became "disinhibited." He was overly friendly with strangers on the street, sometimes frightening them. As his illness progressed, he loudly proclaimed his religious beliefs at restaurants and inquired into those of other patrons. He refused to take custom orders from clients, insisting instead that his vision for making a piece of furniture was better. He had only a few customers left as a result. This disinhibition occurs when connections within the frontal lobes — our seat of judgment and social decorum — erode. Interestingly, such disregard for rules and safety is also a normal phase in teenagers as their frontal lobes develop.

Even so, Dave had a wonderful quality of life. A divorced father of two, he lived in his own home in New Jersey, continued to work on carpentry projects in his backyard workshop, and regularly drove to my office.

Three years after his diagnosis, his sons informed me that Dave had started to consider stop signs as suggestions rather than as essential rules of the road. This was a progression of his disinhibition, but a dangerous one rather than the earlier merely annoying or embarrassing manifestations.

Learning that Dave was ignoring stop signs on a regular basis, I wrote to New Jersey's Department of Motor Vehicles and had his license suspended. Dave came into my office furious.

"What did you do that for, Doc?" Dave yelled, but he was laughing at the same time. He then said, mock threateningly, "I'm going to break your arm!"

"If you were driving, I would feel unsafe on the road," I explained firmly, even as I couldn't help being amused by his approach. "I'm very sorry to have done this to you, because you know I really want you to stay independent. However, it's clear at this time that you are no longer a safe driver."

"I promise I'll stop at stop signs," Dave replied.

"I believe you have every intention of doing that, Dave," I told him. "And I am very unhappy about having to do this, but I really cannot let you drive anymore."

Eventually Dave agreed with me. "I know you're right," he said, letting out a big laugh. "But that doesn't mean I don't still want to break your arm!"

After Dave's license was suspended, his brother would drive him into the city. Every time Dave came to see me, he made a point of complaining about not being able to drive and telling me how much of a stick-in-the-mud I was. Even so, he continued to follow my instructions and did not get behind the wheel again.

Every so often, there are patients in my

practice like Dave, and I have to insist that they stop driving. More commonly, though, my patients continue to drive despite a diagnosis of dementia. By the time most people with Alzheimer's or other dementias get their diagnosis, they have probably been driving for more than fifty years. Driving is a part of the fabric of their brain and not something that they have to deliberately think about. It's an automatic skill, much like hitting at bat was for Yogi Berra. "I can't think and hit at the same time!" he famously quipped.

So, until drivers with Alzheimer's either decide to stop driving on their own or start having small mishaps, like clipping a parked car or a mailbox, I believe it is best to leave their car keys with them. In my experience, patients exhibit early warning signs well before a significant accident. When those signs emerge, I have a discussion with them about stopping driving. Interestingly, about 20 percent of the women patients in my practice (and to this date, none of my male patients) reduce or stop driving on their own, because they feel "anxious" and "not sure" of themselves.

Alternatively, patients and families may choose to take a more objective route and have an assessment by an occupational driving rehabilitation specialist, who puts the patient through a simulated driving test. I don't often prescribe this, because most patients get angry and refuse to take it. But sometimes it's the only way to convince patients of the importance of giving up the car keys. Even after failing a test, some patients continue to drive, and that is when more extreme measures need to be adopted. Happily, this is a rare occurrence.

DRIVING DRUNK WITH DEMENTIA

It's also important to keep in mind that some patients' driving difficulties may not be from dementia at all. Take, for example, my patient Georgina. A retired schoolteacher in her sixties, she lived alone in the outskirts of Westchester County. Georgina described herself as someone with "a passion for vodka," and had been a functional alcoholic for much of her life. She regularly careened over to the liquor store at her local strip mall in her large, late-nineties Chrysler sedan. Because of her Alzheimer's, she was prone to forgetting how much alcohol she had already consumed and began to drink even more. Because she lived alone, there was no one to keep tabs on her, and she insisted on driving everywhere.

Despite her drinking, Georgina never had

an accident. She was, in fact, an excellent driver with a great track record. The problem was that she was becoming a drunk driver without even realizing it, as her memory loss prevented her from realizing how much she'd had to drink.

After various failed strategies, including removing all liquor from her house and telling Georgina not to buy any more, her daughter, Caroline, and I hit upon the idea of surreptitiously diluting her mother's vodka. Caroline lived near enough to visit every few days and would do the "diluting deed" when her mother was not watching. Georgina never guessed that her beverage of choice had been drastically watered down, with dementia likely responsible for her reduced gustatory discernment. Once the vodka was mostly removed from the equation, Georgina, despite her dementia, continued to drive without incident for many years.

Driving is closely tied to one's sense of independence. When you first get your driver's license, it's a big moment. Suddenly you become more of an agent of your destiny. Whether you're taking a road trip or just going to the corner store, the knowledge that you can drive yourself there is a heady one.

I still remember my first solo drive from Brooklyn, where I lived, over the Manhattan Bridge into Chinatown. It was a hot Sunday afternoon, and my border collie mix, Sasha, was in the passenger seat, sitting up, tongue hanging out. The two of us watched as the New York City skyline came into view. That feeling of exhilaration, that freedom, that sense of agency is hard to forget and even harder to give up.

Because driving has so much emotional subtext folded into it, when a patient with Alzheimer's disease can no longer drive, they may experience a level of depression that can be hard for caregivers to fully comprehend. Removing that privilege should not be done lightly.

Ways to Maintain Independence After an Alzheimer's Diagnosis

With good planning, people with Alzheimer's can live functional, independent lives. These tips are directed primarily toward the patient, but are also helpful for caregivers and loved ones to bear in mind.

- Make your wishes about staying at home or moving elsewhere clear.
- Most people can keep driving with Alzheimer's. If there is concern about your ability to drive, you can take a simulated

driving test offered by an occupational driving rehabilitation specialist to assess safety.

- Going where you want, when you want is part of being an adult. When family members get anxious, wearing an ID bracelet can help calm them. Fortunately, they come in chic and sporty styles. If your family is very anxious, consider wearing a GPS tracking device. There are lots of unobtrusive options.

- If you need at-home help to supervise medication, think of it as support to help you stay independent and at home longer.

TREASURE HUNTING

Being in charge of one's finances — deciding what to spend on whom and on what — is another major part of being independent. As with driving, a dementia diagnosis can trigger some knee-jerk reactions; family members may assume that the patient will make poor decisions and take away his or her financial control, even if a patient's spending habits haven't changed. Patients who have been spendthrifts all their lives may find that their freewheeling ways are being curtailed by family members who have different views on money and decide to attribute excessive spending habits to the dementia. Caregivers may want patients to sign over financial authority, a suggestion that many patients, particularly men, find difficult to stomach.

On the other hand, some patients do in fact change their spending habits because of their dementia. They may forget to pay bills or simply leave piles of bills unopened, or pay the same bill several times over. Some may fall prey to con artists calling them on the telephone. On occasion, patients may forget where they have placed various funds or objects of value, something that happens to many of us more often than we would care to admit, as my patient Peter revealed to me.

Peter came to me about his chronic back pain. Although I specialize in memory disorders, I also see patients with other neurologic conditions like migraines, back pain, vertigo, and stroke.

"Maybe my pain is from the work I do," he told me.

Peter had heavy-lidded eyes, a high forehead, and a mischievous smile, all of which conspired to make for atypically dashing good looks.

"What kind of work is that?" I inquired.

"Well," Peter said with a grin, "do you know that you probably have money floating around that you know nothing about? Checks you didn't cash? Money sent to you that you didn't even know about?"

I doubted that it was possible. My bookkeeper kept meticulous records.

"Of course it's possible!" Peter insisted.

He typed my name and information into my computer. Sure enough, we discovered an uncashed check from years ago, which was now in a repository in New York State.

"I am kind of a modern-day treasure hunter," Peter explained, "but no ships or digging for me. I spend my days hunched over a computer and old telephone books. Banks call me when they find big sums of money in their safety deposit boxes and they can't find the owner. It's my job to track the person down.

"I have telephone books from the 1950s on for trying to find people who have never gone online," he continued. "The problem, Doc, is that now that there's all this Alzheimer's going around, there is an awful lot of forgotten money in the banking systems. I'm going to have a banner time in the years to come."

I realized that this made sense. As we get older, if we develop memory problems and begin to suspect that our families would like to oversee our finances, there is even more of an impetus to put away money or to hide it somewhere. This is because money is intrinsically linked to our personal sense of control and independence.

The question is what to do when patients' spending patterns are clearly a result of the dementia. In extreme cases, patients can spend themselves into destitution, although in my experience, the situations usually aren't so dire. I had a patient who repeatedly withdrew money to buy the same pair of shoes. Another ordered magazines from various subscription services, until his entire apartment was overflowing with them.

"Mom has spent hundreds of dollars on bed linen *again,*" the daughter of a patient told me. "I cut off her credit cards, and now she's furious with me. She's screaming at me that she wants her cards back. They are her cards, but I don't want her doing this anymore."

I understood the daughter being upset at yet another unnecessary set of expensive sheets arriving at her mother's house, but I told her that taking away the cards was too drastic. Control over our finances gives us an important sense of agency, which is not something to be casually taken away. "I think the best thing to do is let your mom keep her cards but put a limit on them, so she has a sense that she's still in charge of her own money," I said.

In the end, the patient had a daily spending limit placed on her account. A compromise was struck, so the patient still had some level of financial independence but her assets were better protected. The same type of limits can be put on bank withdrawals.

Sometimes, patients may refuse to cede financial authority to their family members, and in those cases, it can be very difficult to help oversee their finances. In those instances, I ask patients if they will agree to having a bookkeeper or an assistant of their choosing come in and pay bills, couching it from the perspective of independence. Hiring someone to oversee their bill paying instead of having family members do it is often more palatable to patients who see this as less of a financial "takeover" and more as "secretarial." Occasionally, family members resort to legal means to transfer control of finances, which can be traumatic for all concerned. Sadly, this may be the only viable option in cases where patients are not paying utility bills, for example, but refuse to acknowledge it.

Another common issue is hiding items of value. One of my patients hid all of her jewelry in different corners of a large, rambling house in Connecticut. When the house was being sold, her children couldn't find any of it.

"Where is your jewelry Mom?" they would plead.

"It's safe! It's safe!" was my patient's reply. "I've hidden it away."

The children never did find it.

"The new owners of the house are very lucky," her daughters told me. "There is so much treasure hidden there that we'll never see again."

IMPRISONED

Another area of contention can be patients coming and going as they please. "Cynthia is really upset with me," a patient's husband told me one day. "She got lost this summer on her way home from your office. Ever since then, I don't feel I can let her out by herself. Now she says that I'm behaving like her prison guard. She insists that she's an adult and I should treat her as such, but I'm terrified of her getting lost again."

"I understand your fears," I told him. "But Cynthia needs to feel confident enough to go out on her own. The ideal thing to do is to get her a bracelet with your name and number on it, and then let her go out. This leaves a safeguard in place and gives you peace of mind. If she does get lost again, she will surely find her way home."

Another option that allows patients freedom of mobility while keeping caregivers informed is wearing an electronic tracking device. These devices are constantly being updated and new ones are coming on the market, so I suggest that patients and families research the option that best suits their personal style and budget. I recommend choosing a device with both a long range and a long battery life that the patient can wear. The geo-location function in many cell phones can be a good way to keep track of a loved one, but patients may leave behind or lose their phone. That's why I usually recommend a wearable device; it helps ensure they are not easily separated from it.

In situations like Cynthia's, I have discussions with both the patient who is complaining about being surveilled and the anxious caregiver about the patient getting lost, and suggest either an ID bracelet or a tracking device. Patients are nearly always willing to allow one or the other in order to maintain their independence, particularly when I frame it as a tool to reduce caregiver anxiety — which it is. Finally, the Alzheimer's Association has an excellent Safe Return program. The patient is provided with a bracelet and a twenty-four-hour number engraved on it that any Good Samaritan can call to report a lost person.

INDEPENDENCE VERSUS SAFETY

Being in charge of our finances and being able to go where we please when we please are the badges of adulthood. I generally value the patient's need for these important freedoms over the anxieties of the caregiver. Of course, maintenance of these privileges is nearly always associated with some compromise of absolute safety. But think about it: If one values safety more than enjoyment, allowing your kids to go snowboarding or play football may be just as problematic. If caregivers have a good reason to be afraid of a patient overspending, or having a car accident, or getting lost, then some limitations may need to be put in place, but they need to be implemented with sensitivity. It should be clearly understood that the priority is preserving the patient's confidence and sense of control. Lowering the anxiety level of the caregiver is not the primary goal.

For every one of us, including patients with dementia, a sense of independence is crucial for morale. We all like to call our own shots — or at least feel like we are calling our own shots — and no one willingly gives up that inherent right. This is important to keep in mind when dealing with patients on the Alzheimer's spectrum whose sense of competence and self-worth may already be undermined by the diagnosis. In the long run, helping patients maintain a sense of independence pays off in a better quality of life for both patients and caregivers.

Chapter 6
Will I Pass This on to My Children? The Genetics of Alzheimer's — and Paths to Prevention

"Will our daughter get this?" Celia asked me, her brow furrowed with worry as she held hands with her 70-year-old husband, who sat quietly beside her.

I had just shared with them that Celia, a soft-spoken 69-year-old retired journalist, had rapidly progressive Alzheimer's, with mild memory and language impairment and good life skills. The three of us had agreed on a treatment plan, and now, as our meeting drew to a close, Celia fearfully asked the question that was troubling her most. I could see her husband tense up as she did so. Concerned as they were about this new and unplanned future of theirs, they were just as afraid for their daughter.

"There is an increased risk to your daughter," I told them, "but it is a very small one. Given the type of Alzheimer's that you have, with some lifestyle modifications we can actually reduce your daughter's risk to even below that of someone who has no family history of it."

Their relief was almost palpable.

Like Celia, most patients with Alzheimer's worry about the genetic risks they may pass on to their children. Many are already feeling bad about the burden they pose to children because of their illness, and their guilt is compounded by a fear that their children might inherit the genes for Alzheimer's. Many children also worry about their own risk when a parent is diagnosed.

About 95 percent of all Alzheimer's cases are late-onset, with symptoms beginning after age 65, as Celia's had. Most of these cases are "sporadic," which means the disease is not inherited. This type of Alzheimer's is the focus of most of this book, and it is a multifactorial disease, meaning that many factors contribute to the development of the illness. Sixty percent of late-onset Alzheimer's can be prevented by controlling these factors — sometimes it's as simple as adopting a healthful diet, increasing physical activity, and becoming more socially engaged. Children of patients with late-onset Alzheimer's have only a small increased risk when compared with those without a family history of the disease.

Early-onset Alzheimer's, on the other hand, occurs when symptoms appear before age 65 and is much more genetically based and far harder to prevent with currently available preventive options. It constitutes only 5 percent of cases and is also most often sporadic — in other words, it's caused by a mutation in the patient's own genetic makeup, rather than one he or she inherited. However, the children of patients with early-onset Alzheimer's have a 50 percent chance of developing the disease.

Early-onset Alzheimer's cases are also the most rapidly progressive on the Alzheimer's spectrum, although as we saw in Chapter 1 with Jonathan, who was diagnosed at 44 and is still living on his own at 64, this is not always true. Genetic influences are far stronger in such cases, and inheritance is in an "autosomal dominant" fashion, meaning that each child has a 50 percent chance of inheriting the disease from an affected parent. It is important to realize that it's possible — although improbable — for an affected parent to have four children who never develop the disease. Each child inherits the gene randomly, as with a coin flip. Of course it's possible that four coin tosses

come up "heads," but it's statistically unlikely.

EARLY ONSET: THEO'S STORY

Several types of genes lead to the various
subtypes of early-onset Alzheimer's. That
discussion is beyond the scope of this book,
but I would like to talk about one exceptional family's early-onset story. Theo,
Cindy, and Mike were three siblings at risk
of developing Alzheimer's thanks to simple
bad luck in life's genetic roulette.

At age 16, their mother, Patricia, fell in
love with their father, Peter, a very handsome serviceman who had just returned
from the Korean War. At the time, she was
living in an orphanage, where she had been
placed at the age of 3, after the death of her
own mother. (It was the prevailing attitude
of the time that fathers could not raise
young children, particularly girls, on their
own.)

Patricia and Peter married six months
after they met, and they were such an ar-
resting couple that they were featured on
the cover of a national magazine. This was
the happiest time of Patricia's life, and in
the years after the marriage, she gave birth
to their three children — Theo first, then
Cindy, then Mike.

Within a few years, Peter's behavior became erratic. He developed a rapidly progressive dementia that doctors at the time believed was caused by Creutzfeldt-Jakob disease, popularly known as "mad cow" disease. By the time he was in his late thirties, Peter needed help with all daily life skills, including toileting. Raising three young children at the same time, Patricia had no choice but to place Peter in a nursing home. He remained there, mute and bed bound, for a remarkable twenty years until he died at the age of 59. Despite the pressures of raising her children alone, supported only by her job as a day care worker and Peter's government pension, Patricia visited him faithfully every week.

Patricia was effectively a single mother. At first, her little family thrived despite the difficult circumstances — her children grew up, and all seemed well in her world. Her eldest son, Theo, got married and moved away to start a family of his own, getting a job as a driver for a delivery company. But he began to develop behavioral problems at 29, just as his father had before him. Marina, Theo's wife, noticed that he was behaving erratically and experiencing memory problems. Over the next two years, his symptoms got worse, and eventually the

201

delivery company had to lay him off because he was unable to remember how to get to even familiar pickup locations.

A particularly alarming incident spurred the family to action. Theo, Marina, and their young daughter, Molly, went out for dinner at a restaurant one evening. Molly began to cry inconsolably, and Theo picked her up and took her outside to pacify her, as he had done many times before. When he returned a few minutes later, however, he was alone.

"Where is Molly?" Marina asked in surprise. "What have you done with her?"

"I've taken care of her," Theo replied.

"What do you mean, Theo?" Marina asked, beginning to panic.

It turned out that Theo had shut Molly in the trunk of their car, thinking it would soothe her. Marina knew in that moment that something was terribly wrong. Theo was a loving and caring father, and what he did that evening was completely out of character. Marina took Theo to a series of physicians who offered a variety of diagnoses, including depression and epilepsy. This made no sense to the couple because Theo had never had convulsions — he had only become more and more behaviorally "off." Marina and Theo came to see me because I was the new specialist in town and they were desperate for another opinion.

I was a newbie myself, in my first year practicing on my own. I had been trained in the intricacies of making a diagnosis of Alzheimer's disease and was running Long Island Alzheimer's Disease Assistance Center.

I suspected that Theo had Alzheimer's disease, but at the same time I couldn't believe it. I was worried that I was making a diagnostic error.

This can't be, I kept telling myself. *He's only thirty-one, and Alzheimer's is a disease of old age.*

I had Theo go through all the tests that I had recently learned about while completing my subspecialty training in dementia. He had an MRI, an EEG, and a PET scan to look at his brain's use of glucose. I did an extensive laboratory workup and a spinal tap. He had a neurocognitive evaluation that he couldn't quite complete because of the level of his impairment. All the tests pointed to Alzheimer's as the diagnosis.

Puzzled, I did some research to see if I could find any other cases in the medical literature where someone was diagnosed at such an early age. I found just one other patient reported in the world literature younger than Theo, a man diagnosed with Alzheimer's at 24. I still struggled to trust my own judgment, but finally I gave Theo and his wife my opinion — that, implausible as it seemed, 31-year-old Theo had early-onset Alzheimer's disease. Interestingly, neither Theo nor Marina was surprised. I think they had been expecting a drastic diagnosis, based on his rapid decline.

After Theo was diagnosed, his mother, Patricia, having spent years watching her own husband slip away, realized that this was a familial condition. She grew frightened that her other children might soon be afflicted as well. Unfortunately, Patricia was right to be worried.

Around this time, Theo's 27-year-old sister, Cindy, began developing symptoms. Both Cindy and Mike, the youngest at 22, still lived at home with their mother in a modest ranch house in a small New Jersey town. Cindy's case developed rapidly, and soon she was unable to get out of bed. Her mother would climb into bed with her to rock and comfort her like a baby. As Cindy's condition deteriorated, Patricia and Mike's lives increasingly revolved around her needs. Mike watched helplessly as both Cindy and Theo deteriorated. He waited anxiously for the inevitable time when he too would develop the illness. He was in limbo, waiting for the sword of Damocles to fall on his head.

At first, Patricia refused to let me examine Cindy because she had had unpleasant experiences with physicians during Peter's illness. She so detested doctors that I suspect that if Theo hadn't been married, there is a good chance I would not have met any of them. It was because of Theo's wife, Marina, that I met him and subsequently learned about Cindy's condition.

Theo's rapidly progressive, early-onset Alzheimer's left him mute and incontinent within a few years of my diagnosis. Sadly I was not able to help him in any substantive way. Even so, I wanted to examine Cindy and obtain blood for genetic analysis. This was the youngest family in the world with the condition, and I wanted to investigate it as best as I could with the available tools. The results would add to the literature in the field, but I also hoped that we could help Theo's daughter, Molly, if she carried the culprit gene. It took some time and persuasion, but eventually, I earned Patricia's trust. I was able to get blood samples from not only Cindy and Mike, but also from the family of her husband, Peter. It took a great deal of research, but eventually we identified a unique mutation in both Cindy and Theo that had caused their early-onset Alzheimer's and that likely had taken their father from them.

Mike was the only sibling left without clinical signs of the illness. He had spent much of his young adult life acting as a caregiver to his affected siblings, and believed his fate was already etched in stone. Over the several years' span that I spent working with and researching this family, I had developed a fondness for this shy and caring young man. He barely spoke but was devoted to his siblings and his mother. Once in a while, I would get a glimpse of his dry humor and we would laugh together. Did Mike also possess the rogue gene that had wreaked such havoc on his family?

Mike was 29 when he got his results. He had been waiting for this dreaded illness to develop since he was 20. However, we happily discovered that Mike did *not,* in fact, have the mutation that would soon cause the premature deaths of his brother and sister, and I got to make one of the most memorable phone calls of my career. I was extremely excited to let him know the good news, expecting Mike to be relieved, thrilled, and thankful for the information.

Instead, I was met only with silence.

"Are you there, Mike?" I asked.

"Yes," Mike said nonchalantly. "So you are saying I don't have the gene . . ."

I remember being surprised, perhaps even a little hurt. What I had failed to consider was that Mike now had to figure out what to do with the rest of his life. This was a life he hadn't thought he was going to live. Suddenly, he had to come to terms with what he could be without the disease. He was overwhelmed by the possibilities.

Cindy died first, at home with Patricia holding her as she took her last breath. Theo followed a few months later, four years after he had first sought treatment.

Eighteen years have passed since I made that phone call to Mike. I hope he has found happiness and a path in life. I know that wherever he is, he is not suffering from the tragic illness that took his father, his brother, and his sister from him. But when I look back on the case now, Patricia is the one who stands out for me. In many ways she personified motherhood and the face of love and resilience in the presence of overwhelming odds. She decided to speak to me, even though she hated doctors, because she wanted to figure out if there was anything that could be done to save her youngest son. Even though her experience gave new meaning to hard-luck stories, she never complained, and she fought for her children with an awe-inspiring fierceness and determination. To this day, when I am feeling sorry for myself, I think of Patricia's strength and tell myself to snap out of it.

A MULTIFACTORIAL DISEASE

As I mentioned earlier, late-onset Alzheimer's is determined by genetics only to a small degree. One thing that proves this is the fact that if one of a pair of identical twins develops late-onset Alzheimer's, it's statistically more likely that his or her twin will *not* get the condition than that he or she will. This would not occur with a disease that is determined solely by genetics. It is clear that later-life factors (in addition to early-life environment, which is usually similar in identical twins) contribute significantly to whether a person develops clinical evidence of late-onset Alzheimer's.

In 2011 the Alzheimer's Association and the National Institute of Health introduced the concept of preclinical Alzheimer's disease. People diagnosed with this have all the biological markers — brain deposits and brain changes — seen with Alzheimer's, but no change in memory or cognition. This stage can last as long as two decades or more before any symptoms manifest. In fact, patients at this end of the Alzheimer's spectrum may die at a ripe old age without ever developing symptoms. What protects them even as their identical twin brothers and sisters begin to show cognitive loss? What role does genetics play, and how can the environment alter a person's genetic inclinations? Although we don't yet have definitive answers to these questions, it is clear that mitigating risk factors and improving heart health and general fitness prevents many cases on the spectrum.

The Genetics of Alzheimer's

Here is an overview of the modes of inheritance and major genes implicated in Alzheimer's.

Late-Onset Alzheimer's

- Symptoms manifest after age 65
- Common — 95 percent of all cases (of these, 5 percent inherited with family history of late-onset Alzheimer's; 95 percent sporadic — no family history)
- Multifactorial, with genetics playing a small role; 60 percent of cases are preventable
- Course varies dramatically from person to

person — can be rapidly or slowly progressive
- Associated with the APOE4 allele of the APOE gene on chromosome 19

Early-Onset Alzheimer's
- Symptoms manifest before age 65
- Rare — 5 percent of all cases (of these, 10–15 percent inherited with family history of early-onset Alzheimer's; 85–90 percent sporadic or with family history of late-onset Alzheimer's)
- Strongly genetic — 50 percent of children will get the disease; cannot be prevented
- Usually rapidly progressive, although exceptions occur
- Seen with mutations in chromosomes 1, 14, and 21

UNDERSTANDING THE RISK

I like to reassure patients and their families by giving them data from one of the largest studies I have ever done. I looked at more than 5,500 siblings and parents of patients with Alzheimer's alongside age-matched adults who did not have the disease. Presuming that everyone lived to 90 years of age, I found that those with a relative with Alzheimer's had about a one-in-four chance of developing late-onset Alzheimer's, whereas those without an afflicted relative had a one-in-five chance of doing so. In other words, if neither my parents nor my siblings have Alzheimer's (and I live to age 90), I still have a 20 percent chance of getting it. And my friend Kitty, whose mother had Alzheimer's, has a 26 percent chance.

It's worth noting that statistics can be presented in ways that make the odds sound more alarming. For example, in my study, we concluded that someone whose mother had Alzheimer's had a 50 percent increased risk (risk ratio of 1.5) for developing Alzheimer's when compared with someone like me (risk ratio of 1.0), once we had factored in variables that could contribute to the difference, like education.

Similarly, contrast the varying ways in which the statistical results of a large study of identical twins could be reported. The study followed 11,000 sets of twins over the age of 65. One way to report the results would be that 55 percent of one of a pair of identical twins did not develop Alzheimer's, and 45 percent did. Another way to report the results would be that genetic factors were responsible for 80 percent of Alzheimer's cases. Although both these sets of statements are true, the take-home message from each is quite different.

Despite these statistics, I can empathize with children of patients with Alzheimer's when they fear that they too will develop the disease. Although I do not have a first-degree relative with dementia, my mother had a chronic progressive neurologic condition that led to her death after a decade-long struggle. As I watched her grow ill, even as her spirit burned undiminished, I was inspired to explore all possible avenues to maintain her quality of life. In fact, she was the reason why I began to explore neuromodulation techniques like transcranial magnetic stimulation (TMS). Although it was too late for TMS to benefit my mother, I know she would be happy that it is benefiting others. I owe much of my drive and success to her, but my awareness of her illness also makes me worry whenever I have a minor fumble.

Every time I stumble or choke on water, a niggling part of my brain lights up with alarm. *Is this the first sign?* I think. I realize that we all stumble on uneven sidewalks. And I know that when one has a tendency to talk and drink at the same time, as I do, there may be occasional coughing spells. What's more, as a neurologist, I am aware that my risk of inheriting the genes of my mother's illness is minimal. But the brain is not a rational organ — at a deep, highly hardwired, and very primitive level it is ruled by emotion. Of course we forget things sometimes — in fact, we are wired to forget, just like we are wired to stumble or choke occasionally. But when there is a family history of Alzheimer's, ordinary acts of everyday forgetfulness acquire an ominousness that can be hard to shake.

When I meet patients for genetic counseling, I try to be sensitive to their fears, both rational and irrational. But I also tell them that they can do things that will actually reduce their risk for developing Alzheimer's to below that of their peers whose parents did not have the illness. In addition to lifestyle, diet, amount of exercise, and conditions like high blood pressure and diabetes, one's level of educational and occupational engagement seem to make a difference. All these variables influence two key factors that ultimately determine the clinical presentation of Alzheimer's: brain reserve and cognitive reserve.

As I mentioned in earlier chapters, brain reserve is a physical measure of the number of brain cells. The larger the number of cells, the larger the brain is physically and the greater the brain reserve. Strokes and head injuries eat into brain reserve, reducing the number of cells. Cognitive reserve, on the other hand, measures the number of connections between nerve cells and the robustness of the brain circuits; in other words, it's about how much we use the brain we have.

Formal and informal education increase cognitive reserve, as do activities as disparate as Sudoku and fox-trotting, by increasing nerve cell sprouting and the connections between cells, much as a bare, dying tree bursts into lush life with the right mixture of soil, water, and weather. Our 80 billion-plus neuronal trees flourish and are kept strong by good blood flow and a healthy lifestyle, even in the face of disease. Inactivity and isolation reduce cognitive reserve, withering neuronal sprouts and weakening vital brain circuits. High blood pressure, diabetes, and heart disease can all lead to reduced brain blood flow, which has a negative impact on both brain reserve and cognitive reserve.

To avoid abnormal plaque pathology and stay on the preclinical end of the Alzheimer's spectrum in the event of such pathology, we need to safeguard brain reserve by protecting our brains from injury and increase cognitive reserve with lifestyle changes.

XAVIER'S QUEST TO PREVENT ALZHEIMER'S

"I'm worried that I'm becoming like my dad," said Xavier, a no-nonsense 50-year-old businessman and the son of one of my patients. "Like him, I find myself forgetting. I need to know if I am developing Alzheimer's so I can plan for the future. I also remember you said that sixty percent of Alzheimer's like the type my father had can be prevented. We need to come up with a game plan."

I had met Xavier when he accompanied his father on a visit to my office the year before. I had diagnosed his dad with a mixed dementia arising from both Alzheimer's and small strokes.

"Don't get me wrong: I never had a good memory to begin with," Xavier continued. "I've never been good with names or faces, but lately it seems to have gotten a lot worse. The other day I blanked on my business partner's name, and we've been together for twelve years. I am concerned, especially given my dad's condition."

At the time, Xavier was experiencing other significant sources of stress as well. His adult son had recently been killed in a car accident, which had, naturally, been devastating. The loss had strained his relationship with his wife.

"Of course, this affects my overall state of mind. It's hard to concentrate, because I am so sad," he said. Furthermore, Xavier was overweight and had high blood pressure, high cholesterol, and chronic insomnia, sleeping only about five hours a night.

I had Xavier go through a testing protocol that evaluated all of his risk factors for dementia, specifically looking for factors that contribute to the disease that we could prevent. We checked his laboratory data for his cholesterol, diabetic risk, thyroid function, stroke risk indices, and genetic risk for Alzheimer's. Because his wife had complained about his excessive snoring, he underwent a sleep study. He had a brain MRI to look for potential problems with his brain circulation. He also underwent a neurocognitive evaluation, so we could get an accurate measurement of his brain's functional abilities and establish a baseline for future comparison.

The results of this thorough evaluation were exactly what we needed to get Xavier the tailored help he required to prevent Alzheimer's. His sleep study showed that he had sleep apnea, a condition that can be caused or worsened by weight gain. Patients with the condition stop breathing while sleeping, sometimes hundreds of times a night, for anywhere from a few seconds to a minute, and this temporarily deprives the brain of oxygen. I thought Xavier's sleep apnea was making his high blood pressure, memory loss, and depression worse. He began wearing a special mask to bed, which allowed him to get several hours of uninterrupted sleep each night for the first time in years. Not only did this reduce his risk for developing Alzheimer's by helping to control his blood pressure and alleviating his depression, but wearing the mask also afforded him better-quality sleep, which further reduced his blood pressure and depression. His brain MRI revealed that he'd had a few small strokes. This surprised him but not me, because such small strokes are not uncommon in those with high cholesterol and hypertension. Like most patients, Xavier didn't even know he had had them, which unfortunately kept him from preventing new ones. These very small strokes, if allowed to increase in number over time, can eventually cause serious problems with thinking and mobility and may even lead to dementia, as was the case with Xavier's father. I told Xavier that controlling his hypertension and cholesterol was essential. Xavier began a heart-healthy, Mediterranean diet and started a program of forty-five minutes of aerobic exercise three times a week. In conjunction with his internist, I also optimized his medication regimen to make sure that his blood pressure and cholesterol were under control. All of this — better blood pressure and cholesterol control, prevention of more mini-strokes, a brain-healthy diet, and aerobic exercise — reduced his risk for Alzheimer's.

His neurocognitive performance showed some mild memory loss and trouble with language, but I thought that was likely related to anxiety and stress rather than from pathology on the spectrum. He began taking an antidepressant under the supervision of a psychiatrist. Xavier was a type-A person — hypercompetitive and driven to succeed — and because he was a man in his fifties, this put him at risk for cardiac problems like heart attacks. I suggested he and his wife talk with a counselor to address the problems they were having over the loss of their son, and encouraged him to begin some type of meditation or relaxation therapy. Reducing stress and anxiety is also important for keeping the brain healthy and functional.

Unable to embrace meditation — "I am just too hyper to relax like that, I guess" — Xavier took up running, which he found to be calming. It had the added benefit of increasing brain blood flow and getting Xavier in better shape, which is also helpful in preventing Alzheimer's. His genetic testing showed that he had one of the E4 variants of the APOE gene associated with a higher risk for developing Alzheimer's. I discussed this with Xavier, and it motivated him to be even more committed to his prevention strategies. I told Xavier that with the kind of modifications he had embraced, it was highly likely that we could prevent him from developing Alzheimer's. Even if he were to develop the brain pathology associated with Alzheimer's, he could remain at the preclinical end of the Alzheimer's spectrum without functional problems.

Xavier has done well in the years since we instituted his prevention regimen. He is back at his college weight, and in fact he says he is in better shape than he was then. He has become fit enough that his sleep apnea resolved and he no longer needs a sleep mask. As his fitness improved and his sleep apnea disappeared, his blood pressure normalized and he was able to stop taking those medications.

Xavier is a success story for many reasons, but especially because he had the courage to challenge what he thought was an unchangeable destiny.

Although he was proactive about assessing his risk for dementia, his approach was atypical. More often than not, children of patients with dementia worry about developing it but don't do anything to try to prevent it. I think the fear of a diagnosis as well as an assumption that the condition can't be prevented keeps them from making an appointment, but such fear is misplaced, as we saw with Xavier. Inheriting Alzheimer's is not as inevitable as many patients and their families seem to think — especially when prevention strategies are employed. It's thought that about 60 percent of all late-onset Alzheimer's cases are actually preventable with widely available therapies and relatively simple lifestyle modifications.

Because so many modifiable elements go into the development of clinical Alzheimer's, it's my experience that at-risk children can significantly reduce their chances of getting the disease by embracing healthier lifestyles and practices. Ideally, women and men should have neurocognitive baselines established at age 50, just as we have baseline bone densities and colonoscopies. This allows for the creation of simple yet tailored programs to improve cognitive health and stave off decline. In addition, there is a baseline for performance comparison down the road, should any cognitive concerns arise. Many neuropsychologists offer such testing in an outpatient setting. The tests can be time-consuming and expensive, and insurance companies may sometimes not reimburse the costs for them, but I believe the long-term benefits are significant.

Although the genetics of Alzheimer's is complex, the good news is that the most common type of Alzheimer's — the late-onset version — is the one most amenable to prevention by the adoption of effective strategies. I advocate a practical approach to prevention for children of patients but also for those of us without a family history of Alzheimer's. In one way or another, Alzheimer's disease will very likely affect either us or someone dear to us at some point in our lives.

CHAPTER 7
DO I FACE SPECIAL CHALLENGES AS A WOMAN?
GENDER AND ALZHEIMER'S

Women bear a disproportionate burden when it comes to Alzheimer's disease, both as caregivers and as patients. Women make up two-thirds of informal (unpaid) caregivers of Alzheimer's and dementia patients. Wives are more likely to provide care for husbands than vice versa, and daughters are more often caregivers than sons. Women provide more intensive care, with five women for every two men providing 24/7 caregiving, and as a result, more women suffer from caregiving-related depression. There is also more of a professional toll on women caregivers, with 20 percent going from full-time to part-time employment, compared with 3 percent of men. Paid caregivers are also far more likely to be women than men.

Furthermore, women are more likely to suffer from Alzheimer's, making up two-thirds of the patients in the United States.

The fact that women live on average five years longer than men accounts for some of this increased risk, but being female in and of itself confers an additional risk. Much of this increase in risk occurs later in life, generally after the age of 80. Although there are several theories about why women may be at higher risk, there is no definitive answer yet. Possibilities include differences in educational attainment, the interaction of hormones — particularly estrogen — with genes, and the greater cardiovascular mortality of younger men compared with younger women. This last factor means that the older male survivors have healthier cardiovascular systems than their female counterparts, reducing a major risk factor for developing Alzheimer's.

In this chapter, I focus on an area that I have been particularly sensitive to in my years of practice and one to which I have devoted many years of research: the misdiagnosis of women, owing both to menopausal symptoms mimicking Alzheimer's and diagnostic bias on the part of the physician. This topic is rarely covered in books on memory loss, and it can have devastating, long-term repercussions for the women involved.

Menopause as a cause of cognitive loss is

underrecognized, leading to unneeded alarm in women going through the menopausal transition in their forties and fifties. Some women going through menopause experience changes in their memory and their ability to multitask and find words. Understandably, their anxiety levels soar because they worry that they are developing Alzheimer's. When these women come in for an evaluation, I am able to reassure most of them, based on results of my testing. Sometimes, though, as in the case of Catherine, whom we met in the first chapter, a thorough evaluation does reveal Alzheimer's. A second issue — one that, fortunately, is less common — is physician bias in diagnosing diseases in women, whether it's heart disease or Alzheimer's. I am concerned that both of these issues, gender based as they are, add even further to the tremendous burden that women already face with regard to Alzheimer's.

MENOPAUSE-RELATED COGNITIVE CHANGES

I first became aware of the unusual challenges that women with cognitive problems face early in my career, when I made a misdiagnosis that dramatically changed my career trajectory. As has often been the case in my practice, a patient inspired the change.

Grace arrived in my office at Columbia University's Alzheimer's Center with her four strapping sons. She was visiting New York City from Brazil, not only to shop but also to have a thorough neurologic workup. "I've lost my mind!" she declared.

Grace was a blond 58-year-old who had had every kind of plastic surgery you could think of. Despite this, her natural beauty still shone through; she had been a pageant queen in her younger days. All of her sons looked like movie stars. When they all crowded into my small office, I felt decidedly unglamorous in my large lab coat.

After an extensive clinical and laboratory evaluation, the center's diagnostic team — made up of neurologists, psychiatrists, neuropsychologists, and social workers — discussed Grace's case. A diagnosis by consensus allows input from multiple perspectives and usually helps prevent clinical errors in decision making. When such multispecialty feedback is available, it can be invaluable in both learning opportunities for all the participants and improving diagnostic accuracy. As a team, we collectively arrived at a diagnosis of Alzheimer's disease. When I told Grace, she wept in my office, comforted by her ever-present sons.

To combat the disease, I put her on medication, including estrogen. At the time, research had indicated that women bene-fited from the use of estrogen in the treat-ment of Alzheimer's, and I thought it was worth trying.

Six months later, Grace returned to my office from Brazil. She burst through the doors on a warm December day, wearing a crisply tailored jacket with crested gold braids over the breast pocket. Surrounding her, as ever, were her four sons, each a bodyguard in his own right.

"I'm cured!" Grace happily declared. "My Alzheimer's is gone!"

"What do you mean?" I asked, thinking to myself that this couldn't be true because although the course of Alzheimer's can be stayed, it is not yet curable.

"I'm cured!" Grace beamed. "Ask my sons!"

"Mom is back to normal," one of her sons said, and they all nodded in agreement with their beloved mother.

Once again, we put Grace through an extensive series of tests. To my great sur-prise, she was correct: All of her deficits had completely resolved, and she no longer had any signs of memory loss or cognitive problems.

How is this possible? I wondered.

Confused, I went back and looked at Grace's case history and the extensive evaluations we had done on her, including a spinal tap. Reexamining her files, I realized that her cognitive changes could have been caused by menopause. At 58, she was atypical in that she had undergone menopause later than most women, ceasing to menstruate just one year before. Interestingly, it was only upon questioning her on her return, after her seemingly miraculous cure, that I discovered this fact. At the time of the initial evaluation, her menopausal history had been of no interest to me and I did not make note of it.

By putting her on estrogen, I had hoped to alleviate her Alzheimer's symptoms, but I ended up with a greater benefit: curing her of the real cause of her cognitive complaints, which was related to declining estrogen levels, another condition entirely. Subsequently, over years of experience, I have learned that estrogen replacement helps with cognitive symptoms in some but not all patients with menopause-related memory loss. Serendipity had been at work in this particular case.

I thank Grace for her role in prompting me to consider an important cause of cognitive change in middle-aged women and for the research I have subsequently done in this area. Because of Grace, my management of women with memory disorders has changed for the better and is much more comprehensive today.

KAY'S "ALZHEIMER'S"

Kay was a patient who many years later benefited from my diagnostic error with Grace. She was a senior hospital administrator and the wife of an ophthalmologist. In her late forties, Kay began to have trouble managing at work. She was having difficulty finding words and could no longer make appointments or multitask. Terrified that something was seriously wrong with her, she sought medical attention and was eventually referred to the Alzheimer's center at a university hospital.

Kay was carefully followed over two years at the center, during which her symptoms worsened. This was borne out by objective cognitive testing. A diagnosis of Alzheimer's disease was made.

Shortly afterward, Kay came to see me for a second opinion upon the referral of her gynecologist, who was aware of the cognitive changes surrounding menopause. At this time, she was 52 years old. After I performed cognitive testing, I found that the pattern of her memory loss was typical of menopause-related cognitive loss, and not of Alzheimer's disease.

I reviewed Kay's extensive medical records from the Alzheimer's center and, not surprisingly, found no mention of her menopausal symptoms. Generally, neurologists and memory disorder specialists do not make note of menstrual histories unless a woman is suffering from conditions such as migraines and seizures known to be affected by hormone levels.

I informed Kay and her husband of my diagnosis, and was met with understandable skepticism mingled with cautious hope. Kay had been carefully followed and diagnosed by a respected senior physician in the field of memory disorders. How sure was I of my diagnosis, they wanted to know. My diagnosis obviously had vastly different prognostic implications than a diagnosis of Alzheimer's. I said I was confident in my assessment but understood their confusion, and I went over my research with them to address their questions.

Unfortunately in the several months since she had received her Alzheimer's diagnosis, both Kay and her husband had changed their perspective on their future and Kay's competence. Ever the perfectionist, Kay had lost nearly all confidence in herself. Much like Ruth from Chapter 3, whose Parkinson's disease symptoms had been misdiagnosed as Alzheimer's, Kay had begun to behave like a patient with Alzheimer's. In addition, in light of her diagnosis, her husband had persuaded her to apply for disability benefits. The application had been quickly approved, confirming for Kay her own deep-seated fears of the level of her dysfunction.

Kay was particularly distraught about the Alzheimer's diagnosis because she had a 10-year-old daughter and was terrified that she would miss important milestones in her daughter's life. She was correctly aware that Alzheimer's that manifests before the age of 65 is usually an aggressive type on the disease spectrum, progressing rapidly to debilitating loss of function within a decade.

"I want to see my daughter get married," Kay told me. "That's the thing I want more than anything else in the world."

I told Kay I believed she would be fine and that I didn't think she had dementia at all. But as much as Kay wanted to believe me, she still felt that she was functioning poorly, and she had the other physicians at the memory disorders center and the insurance company telling her she had Alzheimer's.

Fast-forward five years to 2012, when a new test came on the market that assessed for plaques in the brain: the Amyvid scan. Kay returned to see me. I was happy to see that her condition had remained stable — in fact, she appeared to have improved significantly. She asked me if she should take this new test, and I could almost feel her trembling trepidation mixed with hope. What if, as she secretly hoped, she didn't have Alzheimer's? What if, as she greatly feared, the tests confirmed what everyone else but me had been saying — that she had it?

The test was performed, and Kay had no evidence of plaque in her brain. Here she had been thinking she had Alzheimer's for many long years, when, in fact, she did not. All she had had was menopause-related memory loss that had since improved.

Kay was very relieved. However, she had been living with the label of Alzheimer's for years and collecting disability instead of working. Those years had forever changed her, as they had Ruth. Kay had spent years cross-examining herself and all of her daily minor memory lapses — the kind we all experience — which had left her self-confidence in tatters.

Kay's case illustrates a situation specific to women with memory loss, with her cognitive problems arising from the meno-pausal transition. Her gynecologist was aware of these changes, prompting her refer-ral to me. Her other neurologist, despite be-ing experienced in memory disorders, was not attuned to menopause as a cause for cognitive loss and diagnosed Kay with Alz-heimer's. Obviously, menopause-related cognitive loss needs to be better known in the memory disorders community. Getting a history on changes in menstrual cycle should be as automatic as getting a history on head injury or stroke in women seeking cognitive evaluations. Barbara Sherwin at McGill University was the first researcher to discover this link in 1988, and yet, nearly three decades later, despite much research confirming a link between menopause and cognitive changes, this diagnosis is not routinely looked for or considered by ex-perts. This can be particularly problematic for the adult daughters of patients with Alz-heimer's, who may be more vigilant about their memory lapses than average middle-aged women. They notice cognitive changes associated with menopause, worriedly misattribute them to early Alzheimer's, and seek help, possibly acquiring an erroneous diagnosis.

COUNSELING CLAIRE

Claire was one such at-risk daughter who came to me for genetic counseling. An energetic, bubbly woman of 50, Claire had been an acquaintance for many years. She worked as a secretary at a real estate firm, and I knew she spent a fair bit of time caring for her parents, who lived several hours away.

Claire's mother was 82 with Alzheimer's and doing poorly, and her father, at 86, was more frail than he would admit. Claire had occasionally asked me for advice on her parents' care over the years. Even though I was not her mother's neurologist, I was happy to help. I had suggested that she help them stay in their own home by hiring a live-in companion, which she was able to do with their small pensions. Her parents had lived in the same small town all their lives. Claire had initially wanted to move them closer to her, but I thought that would be disruptive and detrimental to their health.

One day Claire called me in a panic.

"I think I have it," she said. "I have Alzheimer's."

She told me what was happening. "I used to remember our clients' names, but now I keep forgetting them. I used to be able to memorize a five-broker appointment schedule, but now it's like the appointments have been erased from my head. I'm freaking out. I need to come in and see you. You've got to tell me if I am going to end up like my mother."

Claire came to my office and we continued the conversation.

"I'm so like my mother," she explained. "We look alike, we're both allergic to shellfish, we both have the same temperament — we fly off the handle easily. Who's going to take care of me? I don't have kids."

Upon closer questioning, I discovered that Claire had recently been going through perimenopause. Her periods had become less frequent over the last year. She had gone to her internist, who performed blood work and told her that notwithstanding her symptoms, the tests revealed that she was not yet menopausal. I explained to Claire that, given the irregularity of her previously regular menses and the fact that she was beginning to have night sweats, it was likely that she *was* going into menopause, despite the test results. "Clinical symptoms are more sensitive indicators of impending menopause than lab tests," I added.

Claire underwent a neurocognitive evaluation that I had specifically adapted for testing women like her. Her neurological and general medical examination was normal. Her neurocognitive results showed trouble with memory and language, which can also be seen early in the course of Alzheimer's disease — one reason why Kay was erroneously diagnosed with Alzheimer's. However, the pattern of her test results in its entirety was consistent with menopause-related cognitive loss. I was able to reassure Claire that her symptoms were likely from menopause and not from dementia.

After consulting with her gynecologist, I gave Claire the option of either going on hormone replacement or treating her symptoms with brain exercises. Claire was frightened of hormones. She recalled at least two people in her life who had developed breast cancer after taking hormones. I tried to reassure Claire that her chances of developing breast cancer with hormone replacement for the first few years of treatment were the same as the chances for women not on hormone therapy, but she didn't buy it.

"What about strokes?" she asked me.

"Isn't there a risk for blood clots too?"

I had to admit that there was, in fact, an increased risk for blood clots on hormone replacement.

"And the memory problems? Are you sure they'll get better with hormones?"

"No," I said. "We can't know until we try. Some women improve with hormone replacement, but others don't."

Claire decided against hormone replacement, but began a course of weekly tailored brain exercises to improve her memory and word retrieval. After six months, she thought she had reached the stage where her functioning had returned to normal, and she has been fine in the many years since.

In other cases like Claire's, I have prescribed donepezil, a medication used with Alzheimer's because the underlying neurochemical deficit in menopause-related cognitive loss is the same. In both Alzheimer's and menopause there is a reduction in acetylcholine in the part of the brain that deals with memory. In my research and clinical experience, donepezil has benefited women with menopause-related cognitive loss.

Some women may not notice improvement in their cognition when they begin treatment, whether with hormones or with donepezil. However, hormone replacement is remarkably effective in treating the night sweats and hot flashes that prevent a good night's sleep. Because restful sleep is a key factor in good memory functioning, even when hormone replacement therapy does not help directly with cognition, it does so indirectly by allowing better sleep. (Studies have found that poor sleep as well as use of common sleep aids like diazepam [Valium] increases the risk for Alzheimer's by as much as 50 percent, so I never prescribe such medications in my practice.)

In Claire's case I was happy to reassure her, reduce her level of stress, and allow her to continue to be an effective caregiver to her parents. I was also glad that Claire now had a cognitive baseline, so that years from now, if she were to have memory problems that she thought were progressive, she would have a comparison. I was grateful that Claire's story had evolved so differently from Kay's, thanks to my long-ago encounter with Grace and the pioneering research work of psychologists like Dr. Sherwin.

PHYSICIAN BIAS IN DIAGNOSING WOMEN

Although I was always aware of the potential for bias to influence diagnosis in patients who happened to be women, my patient Rosa's case was an eye-opener. Until then, most cases I encountered where a woman's symptoms were misdiagnosed were linked primarily to physicians' lack of awareness of a condition specific to women, such as menopause-related memory loss. At other times, the way female patients exhibited an illness led to the misdiagnosis. For example, the fact that women on the Alzheimer's spectrum often show higher levels of anxiety and depression sometimes leads to a diagnosis of a psychiatric disorder instead of an accurate diagnosis of dementia. Even in cases where my women patients who were subsequently diagnosed with life-threatening encephalitis or stroke were sent home with anxiety medication from the emergency room — parenthetically, I cannot recall a single case of a male patient with a similar story in my practice — there was nearly always an at least partially plausible reason why such an error in judgment occurred. There was no such excuse with what happened to Rosa.

Rosa was the sister of my patient Carmen, who had died eight years previously. When Carmen's daughter, Valeria — Rosa's niece — called me one day, I was pleasantly surprised.

"How are you?" I asked. I hadn't heard from Valeria in years. Her mother had been my patient when I was a young neurologist. Every so often, family members of long-gone patients will call me just to say hello. I cannot convey how much I love getting such calls and how much they mean to me. It is wonderful to hear how members of the patient's family are doing and to reminisce with them, bringing back shared memories, both sad and happy. But Valeria had a more immediate and serious reason for getting in touch.

"I'm good, thank you, Dr. Devi," she replied, "but I wanted to talk to you about my aunt. I think she has the same problem that my mother did."

My mind flew back to Valeria's mother, Carmen, whom I remembered well, as hers had been a difficult case to diagnose. When she first came to see me, Carmen was a compact 58-year-old who worked in the administrative department of the school system but had developed progressive problems functioning there. She could no longer type well and kept making mistakes. Even though she'd been at the same office for nearly thirty-five years, she was having difficulty recognizing her colleagues.

"I'm not sure what's the matter with me,"

Carmen said the first time we met at the memory disorders center where I worked at the time. "I feel like my mind isn't my own anymore . . ."

After her workup, Carmen was diagnosed with an unusual form of dementia called corticobasal degeneration. In this dementia, there may be early difficulty with awareness and movement of a single limb, and possible Parkinsonian features — like rigidity and slowness — in addition to later-onset cognitive loss. I prescribed medication, none of which was very effective, because corticobasal degeneration is generally aggressive.

As Carmen's condition deteriorated, I asked her whether, at the time of her death, she would be willing to have her brain autopsied. Carmen readily consented.

"I want to be able to help my daughter," she said. "I only have one child, and if there's anything I can do to help you doctors figure out what's happening, it'll help my daughter too."

After Carmen's death, which unfortunately happened within four years, we autopsied her brain. I discovered that she did not have the unusual dementia we had diagnosed. It turned out that Carmen was on the Alzheimer's spectrum, but with an aggressive, atypical type of disease. Her symptoms were so unusual that, without the advanced plaque-scanning technology that we now have available, corticobasal degeneration had seemed a more plausible diagnosis.

On the phone with Valeria, I was very sorry to hear that her aunt Rosa was dealing with similar problems. I knew Rosa from the years I had taken care of her elder sister, when she often accompanied Valeria and Carmen on the visits to my office.

"Bring her in right away," I instructed.

Rosa came in to see me within a week. At 55, she was a few years younger than Carmen had been when I had diagnosed her. She worked in the same school building where Carmen had worked. She had never married, instead devoting herself to bringing up Valeria with her sister. Rosa was happy to see me, but I could tell immediately that she was anxious.

"I don't want to end up like my sister," she told me, smoothing down her wavy hair nervously. "But I'm worried that the same thing is happening to me."

"I can't believe it," Valeria added. "Rosa has been my second mom my whole life. How could this happen to her too?"

I examined Rosa and, after putting her through a series of tests, reached the sad conclusion that she was, in fact, suffering from the same aggressive type of Alzheimer's her sister had died from. I didn't quite know how to break the news to the family. After all, I had made a mistake with Carmen's diagnosis. Although it was clear that Rosa was suffering with something rather grave, I wanted to get a second opinion to be safe.

As luck would have it, the neurology department at my hospital invited me to present an interesting patient at an upcoming grand rounds. Grand rounds are weekly gatherings where patients' cases are presented and their diagnoses discussed by all departmental physicians — in my case, all the neurologists on staff at the hospital. Discussing patients at these rounds can be both convivial and contentious, but it's always a learning experience. It's a big honor to be asked to present, and I thought it would be a wonderful occasion to present Rosa.

Her case was ideal in many ways for this conference. There was a diagnostic question, she was cooperative and willing to be examined, and I had additional verified family history. Even better, the doctor who was coming in to be the expert discussant for grand rounds was an internationally renowned neurologist, Dr. Parker. We were excited that he was coming to share his clinical acumen with us, a tried-and-true method for passing on skills.

I began by presenting Rosa's story in detail to the group of about fifty physicians and students seated in the auditorium. I spoke of the particulars of Rosa's history and examination, as well as that of her sister Carmen, presenting details of the autopsy we'd performed on her years before.

After that, we invited in Rosa, who had been waiting patiently and nervously outside the conference room with Valeria. She was examined by the great Dr. Parker; an éminence grise in his field wearing a red-and-yellow plaid bow tie, he carried himself with erudition, wisdom emanating from his every pore. Dr. Parker did a complete examination of Rosa and asked her a number of questions in a courteous, calm manner.

The audience — myself and other neurologists, as well as medical students — watched raptly. It was a thorough history, during which Rosa softly recounted the details of her story: Yes, she'd been having problems at work; yes, she was having trouble with her memory; yes, she could no longer enter information into her work computer's database; yes, this was exactly like what her sister had; yes, she was scared that she had the same thing.

The neurological exam was similarly thorough, and Dr. Parker carefully demonstrated the following: Rosa had trouble remembering; she could not follow commands — when Dr. Parker asked her to make a fist, for example, she couldn't quite figure out how; she had trouble finding words; she had some generalized slowness; she was also clearly anxious, which wasn't surprising since she was being examined in front of several dozen people she had never met.

After the examination was complete, I escorted Rosa out of the auditorium so that we physicians could discuss her case in private.

"Well . . ." Dr. Parker said, turning to the room.

Everyone waited with bated breath, as did I, hoping against hope that perhaps he had a different diagnosis, despite the fact that I knew he couldn't: Watching Rosa being examined in the spotlight so well and so thoroughly by someone else had been a déjà-vu experience for me. Rosa had the same symptoms as Carmen, the same clear signs, and, I was convinced — now more than ever, after watching Dr. Parker's skillfully obtained history and masterful examination — the same illness.

"It's clear what her diagnosis is," Dr. Parker said.

He turned to look at me.

"It's obvious," he asserted. "Rosa is *hysterical. Hysteria* is the diagnosis." The emphasis is mine — Dr. Parker actually delivered his verdict in a monotonous, matter-of-fact way, as if to underscore his clinical detachment and lack of bias.

I cannot begin to convey how shocked, horrified, and angry I was. My horror only grew as I looked around the room and saw everyone nodding in agreement with Dr. Parker's outrageous diagnosis. The medical students watched and learned.

"There is no evidence of dementia here," he continued. "She is clearly attention seeking. She wants to go on disability, and that's why she's doing this. She knows how to model this illness because she's seen her sister go through it. So of course she started this a bit earlier than her sister. She wants to get a head start on the disability benefits. It's clear to me," Dr. Parker concluded, "that she is hysterical with some malingering for secondary gain."

I was beyond angry. The malingering part was particularly insulting, implying as it did that Rosa was faking her symptoms. At least the hysteria part of his diagnosis, although also insulting, implied that there was an unconscious psychological cause of her symptoms, albeit with a clear gender bias. *Hysteria* is a term coined in 1900 BC — almost 4,000 years ago — to describe inexplicable symptoms in women. It still exists as a diagnosis in the clinical lexicon, but it is rarely found in textbooks anymore. Even if he had attributed Rosa's symptoms to her obvious anxiety, I may have found some way to forgive him.

"But Dr. Parker," I protested, "she failed all her cognitive evaluations. Her sister had autopsy-confirmed, early-onset Alzheimer's, which as you know has strong genetic underpinnings."

"Yes," he said. "That doesn't matter. We can't really prove that this woman isn't mimicking her sister's symptoms, either deliberately or unconsciously or both."

As the conference wound down, I turned to a colleague whose opinion I trusted. We shared patients and would bounce diagnoses off one another other when in doubt.

"Ed," I said, "what do *you* think?"

Remarkably, Ed agreed with Dr. Parker, who had complete sway over his audience's opinion because of his extraordinary reputation.

That day was a learning experience for me, but not the kind I'd hoped for. I learned that despite hearing the same history and watching the same examination, a room full of neurologists could come to vastly different conclusions, based on preexisting prejudices, whether about the patient being examined or about the doctor examining the patient.

After grand rounds, I met with Valeria and Rosa, who were waiting outside the conference room for the verdict.

"What did he say?" they both asked anxiously.

I escorted them back to my office, trying to buy time as I figured out what to say. I didn't have the heart to tell them that in this famous professor's opinion, Rosa was faking her symptoms. I did the best I could to paraphrase the discussion while being honest.

"He thinks," I finally said to Rosa, "that you may be anxious about Carmen and that that is why you are now experiencing these symptoms. He thinks that these symptoms are not from any neurologic problems in the brain."

Rosa and Valeria were speechless. "Of

course she's anxious," Valeria finally said. "Who wouldn't be in her position? But I find it hard to believe that anxiety is the sole cause of my aunt's problems."

"I agree with you," I said. "I don't believe that Rosa's symptoms are from anxiety. Anxiety may be making them worse, but I disagree with Dr. Parker's assessment. It was good to have his opinion, but we are going to continue with our current treatment plan."

They agreed sadly with me. Like me, they'd been hoping for a miracle diagnosis — albeit one that made sense — and a miracle cure. After they left, I wrote an email to Dr. Parker, thanking him for being so thorough in his evaluation and asking whether he had noticed Carmen's small muscle twitches. I pointed out that these kinds of muscle movements aren't seen in "hysterical" patients and that perhaps under the circumstances, he would reconsider the diagnosis. I waited for a response from Dr. Parker but never received one.

Rosa's illness progressed rapidly, as her sister's had before her, and she died within three years. I was unable to help her in any substantive way, just as, sadly, I had failed to help her sister.

Rosa was not alone in being misdiagnosed like this, although her story is the most egregious I've encountered. Too often women get dismissed, their complaints labeled as "hysteria" or written off as anxiety. Compounding diagnostic difficulty, women with Alzheimer's exhibit its signs differently from men, often showing more depression and anxiety-related symptoms. This is all the more reason to do a thorough evaluation with an open mind, rather than make a gender-based, biased clinical judgment.

Thanks to Dr. Parker, a new generation of medical students and some of the neurologists in the auditorium that day will have this ludicrous diagnosis spring to mind when they see a woman with symptoms similar to Rosa's. Because there was no occasion to bring up Rosa's case again in grand rounds, my colleagues did not learn of her "hysteria" progressing to death three years later. The medical students in that room that day went on to become training physicians and are now full-fledged physicians somewhere else, with Dr. Parker's thorough examination and preposterous conclusion a part of their medical education.

In all my years of practice, and after an exhaustive review of the relevant literature, I have found that *hysteria* is a term applied almost exclusively to women. I suppose it shouldn't surprise me — after all, the word was derived from the Latin and Greek root for "womb," and was thought to arise from uterine dysfunction. The notion was of an untethered uterus wandering around the body causing havoc, whether in the form of headache, dementia, or seizures. The Victorian practice of women carrying smelling salts stemmed from the belief that the uterus, disliking the smell, would scuttle back to its place in the nether regions of a woman's body, restoring harmony to her mind and soul.

Sadly for us, *hysteria* is still part of the insurance-reimbursable diagnostic lexicon of today's medicine. The irony in all of this for me is that whereas Rosa had her problems metaphorically attributed to the uterus, Kay had her problems ascribed to a primary brain dysfunction even though they actually arose from a change in her ovarian hormones.

Gender hinders accurate diagnosis more often than I would like, and not just with brain disorders. For example, Marjorie, a patient whom I saw for migraines, raced to the emergency room with chest pains when she was 48, worried she was experiencing a heart attack. To her relief, she was told that she was just experiencing a panic attack and should go home. A couple of weeks later, she returned to the emergency room with yet more chest pains and they told her the same thing: "It's a panic attack — go home."

A day later, she collapsed and was found to have suffered multiple small heart attacks that culminated in a massive one. Tests revealed that she had a rare blood-clotting disorder that predisposed her to these problems. She survived for five years after those events until finally succumbing to her failing heart. I am hard put to think of a circumstance in which a 40-plus-year-old male patient with chest pains would have been told he was having a panic attack and sent home from the hospital.

One of my goals as a doctor is to continue to keep myself aware, and to make others — both physicians and patients — aware of how gender adds certain diagnostic challenges to the practice of medicine. Although the area of menopause-related memory loss continues to be underrecognized in neurology, most obstetricians and gynecologists know about the condition. I'd like to help make more memory experts attuned to this possibility to avoid misdiagnoses such as Kay's and Grace's. It is also essential to be cognizant of any preconceptions that we have as physicians, whether "It's a middle-aged woman — it must be a panic attack" or "An anxious woman? Hysterical, clearly." Recognizing and challenging our preconceptions is necessary if we want to properly care for our patients and not violate the privilege of their trust.

CHAPTER 8
I JUST DON'T CARE ABOUT ANYTHING ANYMORE.
TREATING DEPRESSION AND ANXIETY IN DEMENTIA AND WHAT TO DO ABOUT APATHY

"I just know there's something wrong with me," Della, a 64-year-old dance instructor at a local community center, told me when she visited my office with her two children and her husband.

"We've told Mom that she's overreacting," her daughter said. "She seems totally fine to us."

Della had become increasingly depressed as she noticed subtle changes in her thinking. For most of her life she'd been a vivacious, chirpy woman with sparkling eyes, but in the previous two years she had become more and more withdrawn.

"But I know something's not right with me," Della said. "I think it's why I've been so depressed. I'm not someone who gets depressed easily. My mother died when I was seven, and my father died when I nineteen. But I still managed to finish college and get married. I had several miscarriages before my children came along. All of those things were very sad, but I made it through and became a resilient person. I don't understand why suddenly, now, I've become depressed. I think it's because I'm not able to remember well."

"But there's nothing wrong with you, Mom," her son interjected. "Your memory is the same as mine. You remember everything!"

"But Tommy, I don't," Della insisted. "My mind is not what it used to be. Something's not right. I'm forgetting more and more, and it's making me depressed."

At this point, Della's husband, who had been quiet thus far, spoke up. "Della may have a point," he said. "I've noticed that she's been a little more forgetful. She gets more flustered around holiday dinners when there are extra people to cook for. She wasn't like this before."

It turned out that Della had been developing Alzheimer's disease. During the preceding three years she had experienced mild memory problems, which she couldn't quite articulate. But she had noticed her increasing depression and anxiety, which women with Alzheimer's are more likely to experience than men with the disease. She had felt alone in her condition because she knew there was something ominous in her lapses. She wasn't able to convince anyone, least of all her family, that her memory was failing.

I have found time and again that, like Della, patients early in the course of Alzheimer's are prone to becoming anxious and depressed. And more than half of all Alzheimer's patients suffer from depression and anxiety at some point during the course of their illness. These two symptoms are often linked, with similar underlying neurochemical changes. It is easy to understand why patients would feel depressed and/or anxious when they experience a decline in thinking, functioning, and independence. But some studies have suggested that these symptoms are independent of the pathology of dementia and unrelated to changes in functioning and are caused instead by separate changes in brain chemistry. No matter the cause, it is very important to treat such symptoms. Treatment not only improves memory and attention, but also helps patients become more social and engaged in activities. Patients who previously worried that their cognitive deficits were apparent to others become more relaxed and communicative. This, in turn, helps prevent clinical progression as patients keep using their social and language skills, rather than losing them from nonuse (validating the old "use it or lose it" maxim). Many patients who have become recluses, refusing to leave their home and anxious about socializing, begin enjoying these activities again as treatment takes effect, a process that generally takes about four to six weeks.

I prescribe newer antidepressants, like selective serotonin reuptake inhibitors (SSRIs), to alleviate symptoms. These medications, which we know by brand names like sertraline (Zoloft) and escitalopram (Lexapro), are highly effective in treating depression and anxiety in patients on the Alzheimer's spectrum. The first and most famous drug of this class, fluoxetine (Prozac), is not as commonly used now, as newer iterations have fewer side effects.

"But Doctor," an anxious patient might say upon getting the prescription, "this is a medication for depression. I'm not depressed, I'm anxious. Shouldn't I be taking something like Xanax or Klonipin?"

"You're right, you're not depressed," I agree, "but these medications are also effective at treating anxiety, and are better for a number of reasons. They're not addictive, and they don't interfere as much with your memory or make you as sleepy. The only downside is that it takes a few weeks for them to work, so we have to be patient."

In my practice, I rarely ever prescribe medications of the benzodiazepine class popularly used as anxiety medications — drugs such as diazepam (Valium), clonazepam (Klonipin), lorazepam (Ativan), and alprazolam (Xanax). I will get into my reasons for that later.

I placed Della on a small dose of escitalopram, and over two months, she noticed significant improvement.

"I feel more at peace," Della said. "I'm not as hung up about making a fool of myself when we go out with friends." As her anxiety and depression improved, I added medications to treat her Alzheimer's. I don't like to start multiple medications at the same time because it makes it more difficult to pinpoint the culprit when there is a side effect.

Several months later, at a follow-up visit, Della's son, Tommy, said to me, "It seems like Mom is almost back to her old self. She isn't moping around anymore. She wants to spend time with my kids again."

ANXIETY AND DEPRESSION
MASKED AS IRRITABILITY

In some cases, it's hard to differentiate among depression, irritability, and anxiety. This is not a unique problem, and it holds true for anxious patients with and without dementia.

"She's become so testy lately," Jerry said, complaining about his wife, June, whom I had recently diagnosed with Alzheimer's. "She used to be an angel, and now I can't say a thing without upsetting her. We've had more arguments in the last year than in the entire forty-two years that we've been married. When I ask her what's the matter, she says nothing's wrong. But boy, is she a piece of work these days! I try to calm her down, but that only gets her more upset."

June, who had been listening quietly as Jerry spoke, cut him off before he could continue. "Well, maybe I got tired of being an angel, Jerry, huh? Did you ever think about that?"

When I spoke to June in private, she told me that she was worried that her memory was getting worse and that she was getting more "snappy."

These were classic signs of the depression and anxiety that can manifest early in the course of Alzheimer's. SSRIs are equally effective at treating both, and I used them to treat June with good results. Taking the right medication in such situations can alleviate fraught nerves and tension in both the patient and the caregiver.

Anxiety and depression can present in atypical ways. My patient Betty, 87, with her rather garrulous, acerbic wit, reminded me of Edith Wharton in her heyday. She lived with her husband, who had heart disease. Her anxiety took the form of agoraphobia — she became afraid to leave home, afraid to leave its familiar confines. Before Betty developed Alzheimer's, she had been very sociable and loved going out, meeting friends for lunch and dinner, and attending concerts. After her diagnosis, she became a shut-in and refused to leave her apartment. She was worried about making mistakes in social situations.

Betty became more isolated at home. As time went on, she spent her days plotting to fire her ailing husband's caregivers. She accused them of various imagined misdemeanors, including stealing her underwear and jewelry and flirting with her husband. She frequently questioned their intellectual capabilities. As her anxiety overtook her, Betty became an angry, mean woman.

"My mom used to love everyone who

worked with us," her distraught daughter told me. "She was so kind. I remember years ago, when my nanny was ill, my mom paid for a month-long vacation for her, her husband, and their two children in their home country. She simply believed that they needed it. That's the kind of woman we all knew. I'm shocked at her transformation. It's a good thing my dad's aides knew her before she got like this," she continued, "because I don't think anyone would tolerate this kind of demeaning behavior otherwise."

The good news was that we could treat Betty's anxiety, which was disguised as anger and irritability, with the off-label use of a small dose of the antipsychotic quetiapine (Seroquel). I chose this medication over the SSRIs because I thought it would better address her increasing paranoia. Betty was back to her normal, kind self in just three weeks, with no memory of her past transgressions. This was probably just as well. As I got to know Betty more and more, I realized what a genuinely sweet person she was. She would've been upset to know about her erstwhile nastiness. It was wonderful to find out that she was a generous, big-hearted, funny human being, and not the woman I had first met, made unpleasant by anxiety about her condition, fear of her illness being discovered, and her husband's failing health.

Alzheimer's as a Cure for Anxiety

"My mom was always difficult," the daughter of a patient once told me. "I couldn't get along with her — honestly, nobody could. Nothing was ever good enough for her. But now that she has Alzheimer's, she's become much nicer — even my children have noticed. No more cutting remarks. My father and siblings and I spent our lives trying to please her, and we never made the grade. Now I can do nothing wrong, and she smiles all the time. Maybe she was miserable before and that's why she took it out on us. The change has been amazing!"

The daughter had hit the nail on the head: My patient had suffered from chronic anxiety that had left her critical and angry most of her life, and she became more relaxed and mellow as her Alzheimer's progressed. This is not uncommon. It occurs in about 10 percent of my patients with dementia. Alzheimer's has a mellowing effect, and they become easier to deal with.

SSRIs and Antipsychotics

I am a big advocate of having my patients on the Alzheimer's spectrum live with as little anxiety and as much mental clarity as possible, and when there are drugs that can help achieve that, I embrace their use. My first line of treatment for patients with depression and anxiety, as I mentioned earlier, are the commonly used, nonaddictive antidepressants known as SSRIs. SSRIs are helpful in patients whose anxiety levels are not extremely high and when depression is combined with agitation.

If the patient doesn't respond to SSRIs, or if the symptoms are more intense and there is evidence of psychosis or high levels of irritability, as in Betty's case, then the second line of treatment is antipsychotics. In very small doses, the off-label use of these drugs, including risperidone (Risperidal), quetiapine (Seroquel), and olanzapine (Zyprexa), are helpful in quelling anxiety in patients with Alzheimer's without any risk of addiction and, crucially, without dulling the brain. Issues arise when patients and families, who have no problem with taking the familiar diazepam (Valium) or lorazepam (Ativan), are leery of taking medications associated with psychosis, with its inherent stigmas. Others are fearful of the side effects of these unfamiliar medications.

To make matters more confusing and anxiety provoking, the newer antipsychotics come with a warning specifying that they are not to be used in patients with dementia because of the risk of side effects, including stroke and death. However, at this time, there are no better options for treating some of the troubling behavioral symptoms seen in some patients on the spectrum. In my experience, if used judiciously and with careful monitoring, these new-generation antipsychotic medications are well tolerated and of benefit to many patients who cannot be helped by SSRIs.

I am careful to discuss with my patients and their families any and all risks associated with their prescriptions. I explain the prevailing opinion that these drugs have no place in the management of dementia symptoms, and then reveal why my experience has led me — and many experts in my field — to believe they do. I explain that in my opinion, the benefits vastly outweigh the risks for the patients to whom I prescribe these drugs. I let them know that they will find an insert with a warning when they pick up their medication. I tell them, "When you see the warning, don't get scared and don't throw away the medications, and if you're really nervous, give me a call." Frequently, that is enough to allay fears. But sometimes, despite a preemptive discussion, both patients and families are hesitant to try medications that are clearly labeled as harmful in patients with dementia. Who can blame them?

Once patients have heard a thorough explanation of the pros and cons, more often than not, they begin by trying a small dose and realize how effective it is. The best recommendation is the efficacy of the drug, once it has been tried. Even so, as with all medications, there are sometimes side effects that prevent continued use. The most common of these is drowsiness. It usually occurs early in treatment and resolves with time. As a side note, although I believe in the efficacy of these medications, I am not a proponent of any particular brand.

BENZODIAZEPINES IN ALZHEIMER'S DISEASE

Anxiety is a very treatable condition, thanks to commonly available medications, as we have seen. As I mentioned earlier, I don't prescribe benzodiazepines including diazepam (Valium) or clonazepam (Klonipin). This is because I believe they merely form a Band-Aid over symptoms, rather than addressing the underlying condition. What's more, the use of benzodiazepines in people with Alzheimer's or other types of dementia can increase confusion and memory loss, in the short term and occasionally in the long term as well. Generally, over time, a higher dose is needed to achieve the same effect as tolerance develops, adding to side effects like sedation, which can predispose patients to falls and fractures. And in some cases, there may be a paradoxical response, where the patient becomes *more* agitated as the result of these medications.

Even so, I want to make it clear that many physician colleagues whom I respect have no such reservations and have used benzodiazepines to good effect in their practice. On the plus side, these drugs are fairly powerful, work right away (unlike SSRIs, which take some time to kick in), and can be used as needed, rather than daily. Additionally, patients and caregivers "like" benzodiazepines, as the calming effect is immediately palpable, which is a major reason for their overuse and abuse. Finally, they are free of much of the stigma attached to antidepressants and antipsychotics. Nonetheless, for the reasons I have detailed, I do not prescribe these drugs.

Treating Alzheimer's-Related Behavior Changes

Here's a quick overview of many of the drugs commonly used to treat the behavioral symptoms of Alzheimer's, including depression, anxiety, agitation, aggression, and sleep disorders.

Antidepressants — For treating depression and anxiety I use primarily newer SSRIs, such as escitalopram (Lexapro) and sertraline (Zoloft).

Antipsychotics — For treating severe anxiety and agitation as well as aggression, I use:
• Newer generation medications: risperidone (Risperidal), olanzapine (Zyprexa), quetiapine (Seroquel), aripiprazole (Abilify)
• Older generation medication: haloperidol (Haldol)

Both types have increased risk for mortality and cardiovascular events (1–2 percent).

Anticonvulsants — For treating certain types of anxiety and aggression I use valproic acid (Depakote).

266

Sleep medications — For help with insomnia and sleep-wake cycle disorders, I use:

- Over-the-counter supplements: melatonin, valerian root
- Prescription medications: doxepin, trazadone, ramelteon (Rozarem)

I do not use benzodiazepines — lorazepam (Ativan), diazepam (Valium), alprazolam (Xanax) — in patients with dementia.

"HOME" IS A CONCEPT

Annie was a tiny 86-year-old woman, no more than four feet nine inches, with a shock of white hair that she wore in a prim cut, upturned at the ends. She wore plain little dresses that fell just above her knees, paired with Mary Janes on her feet, which made her look a lot like an earnest, prematurely wizened schoolgirl.

Her daughter had brought her to see me because Annie was becoming increasingly anxious. Annie was living in her home of fifty years with a paid live-in companion, but was up all hours of the day and night, demanding and pleading to be taken "home." No amount of reassurance from her daughter or the caregiver that she *was* home comforted her.

"Take me home!" she kept saying.

It didn't matter how many photographs of happy times in her home they showed her, or how often they reminded her about the tile she had carefully chosen and laid out as the kitchen backsplash. She even remained unconvinced when they showed her the marks she had made on the wall as she proudly kept track of her children's heights as they grew. Annie would listen for a minute, and then get agitated and more insistent on going home.

Home is, for most of us, a place where we feel comfortable, where everything feels familiar and we know where everything is. It's not as much a physical place as it is a concept — a sense of belonging to the place and a sense of being a master of that space. It is a place where we know what things are — yes, that is my bed, this is the kitchen stove. It is a place where we know how to make things work — lift the faucet for water, don't turn it. The toilet flushes with a lever, not a button. Home is ease and safety.

When Annie said she wanted to go home, she was not talking about home in a physical sense but in a psychological sense. Home was a place where Annie felt comfortable in her own skin, in her own surroundings. When people with Alzheimer's don't recognize their home, it means they no longer see the environment in a way that feels familiar. They don't feel effective in that space, and the place doesn't function in a way that is predictable.

So, when Annie's daughter said to Annie, "You are home," and Annie didn't believe it, they were really talking about two different versions of "home."

What Annie hears is "Well, you *are* comfortable!" And she's desperately trying to explain that she's *not:* "This doesn't feel familiar. I am not comfortable. I'm really anxious and scared about all these unfamiliar things happening inside my mind and outside in this space. I want to go home, because home is where I feel safe and warm and everything makes sense."

Both Annie's daughter and her caregiver were frustrated and flummoxed. Annie was uncontainable in her anxiety. In my office, she paced the room, unable to sit still even for a moment. My heart went out to her.

I tried a range of medications, including SSRIs, antipsychotics, and anticonvulsants, both in combination and separately, but nothing worked for Annie. I tried cues that would help orient her, including night-lights and strategically placed family photographs.

I tried having her caregiver tire her out with daytime activities so she returned exhausted to her apartment in the evening to sleep, but that was no help. I even tried introducing an older rescue cat from the shelter, as animals often help with anxiety, but Annie ignored the kitty. (Fortunately, the caregiver enjoyed having it in the apartment.)

Annie paced all day and all night, incessantly, desperate to go "home." She paced so much, she lost weight. Although she recognized her daughter and her son and was pleasant with the caregiver, she had no idea where she was, only that she was not home. The only time Annie stopped pacing was when we gave her enough medication to force her to sleep, but after we did that, she would wake up drowsy and more anxious than ever.

Annie died a year later, pacing till the end, still in a state of agitation and discomfort. I imagined her apartment, with ruts in the parquet floor carved out by her pacing. I was unable to help her. To this day, I wonder what I could have done differently to allow her to have some peace.

Sundowning

Sometimes agitation and anxiety afflict patients only at night, a symptom popularly known as sundowning. This happens when the patient's own internal "body clock" dissociates from the external twenty-four-hour pattern, and can be triggered when external orientation cues, such as sunlight, are removed. Patients may become agitated, irritable, or confused as the evening progresses. Some demand to be let out, or to go home even if they are home, and it is often the impetus for wandering behavior. They may get up and dress for work even though it is 2:00 a.m. and they have been retired for years.

At such times, in addition to medications to help stop the anxiety, the most effective behavioral technique is redirection rather than confrontation. Redirection allows the patient to save face and does not challenge their assumptions about themselves. Better, for example, to be gently told it's a holiday and that's why there's no work today than to be told that you retired fifteen years ago, which may be completely untenable to your sense of yourself as a working person — a sense that's internally true, regardless of the facts. Additional strategies include using orienting cues such as night-lights, keeping evenings peaceful, and maintaining a daily routine.

I believe very strongly in the therapeutic power of animals. I am fortunate in being able to bring my dogs, Lola and Huck, to the office. They not only lower the anxiety levels of all of us who work there, but also reduce the anxiety levels of my patients. Several studies have documented the utility of pets not only in dementia settings, but also in lowering blood pressure and depression. One study of inpatient dementia patients showed lower levels of noise-related agitation and anxiety and lower heart rates when a dog was present. Lola and Huck are a memorable and treasured part of my office team.

On one striking occasion, a 93-year-old patient with Alzheimer's did not recall that her husband of seventy years had died the week before, and told me he was waiting at home. I had last seen her three months earlier and she did not remember me, but she looked around my office and asked, "Where are the dogs?" They were being walked at the time. Another patient who had only the vaguest of ideas who I was nonetheless associated my presence with the dogs, asking me, "Where are your waggy-waggies?"

I have patients who specifically request an

appointment at times when the dogs are in the office and not out on their walk. Often patients who are upset at being at the doctor's dissolve into smiles upon seeing the fluffy Huckmeister and the elegant Ms. Lola. And two or three times a week, I am treated to the sight of a patient sprawled on the carpeted floor with one of the dogs, completely relaxed and at ease. It's difficult to persuade them to disentangle themselves for an exam, but the examination is always better for it. Since I started bringing the dogs to the office, it has been far rarer for me to have to calm a patient down with medication — now about once a year. Before that, despite having a less busy practice, I used medication to calm an agitated patient once every two to three months.

I support patients adopting a cat or an older rescue dog, because animals can both keep their owners more active and offer a sense of connection and intimacy. Younger pups may be too boisterous for my patients on the dementia spectrum.

WHEN THE SHOWER IS A SCARY PLACE

If someone were to fill a pit with snakes and ask you to step into it, you would refuse, even if the person assured you that you would not be hurt. And if that person tried to force you into the pit, you would almost certainly kick, punch, and scream because of entrenched fear and innate instinct about what you *know (or think you know)* is in there. When a person with Alzheimer's refuses to get into the shower, it may be because they are having trouble understanding what the shower is for and that it is water coming down from the showerhead. They become anxious, even if showering used to be a familiar and pleasurable activity.

If you try to force a person with dementia who no longer recognizes water into a full bathtub, you may be unwittingly coercing them into doing something that terrifies them, sending their anxiety levels through the roof. Saying, "It's just water!" to a patient who no longer understands the concept of water is no more reassuring than saying, "It's just snakes." The only way to deal with this situation is to calm the patient's brain. You can start by trying behavioral techniques, including assuming a calm manner, keeping the bathroom well lighted, and introducing the patient gradually into the bathtub, or resorting to a sponge bath if needed. If these strategies don't work, medication to allay anxiety can make a big difference.

Similarly, patients may refuse to get into the car or to change out of clothes that they have worn for several days, because they choose the familiar and comfortable over what they perceive as the lesser known and anxiety inducing. For some people with Alzheimer's, even activities as mundane as walking can be terrifying. Each step can be one of fear and dread, because the ability of the brain to translate a thought into a motor movement — ideomotor apraxia — has gotten lost with the disease. Apraxia can disrupt regular, normally mundane activities when least expected, as the brain is essentially an enormous circuit board with switches and wires, with the switches sometimes failing and other times working well. All this can be confusing and wearying for caregivers.

I remember my first time skiing. I was an adult, and everyone around me already knew how to do it — even the little children on the bunny slope. I was absolutely petrified. I didn't understand the equipment, and the more people told me I could do it, the more anxious I got. I was clumsy and fell often, although the instructor patiently told me it was okay. I kept thinking about how, were she a family member, she would likely be frustrated with my awkwardness and not as gentle; perhaps she would even yell at me to get up and get on with it. I often think about that first day on the slopes when I'm treating patients who are terrified and confused by the things that others around them find so obvious and easy. They understood them once too but the information is no longer consistently accessible.

When you are close to someone, when you have seen them take a million bites before, it's hard not to be frustrated and upset when they are suddenly having trouble eating a sandwich. It can be especially frustrating when their ability appears to come and go randomly, almost as if the patient turns an ability "on" and "off" willfully. A patient who can't remember how to use a fork one day may be perfectly able to do so the next, leading caregivers to think they are faking their symptoms or refusing to use the fork on purpose. Such accusations can make the situation infinitely worse, since stress can increase the patient's inability, whether it's related to walking, speaking, or exiting a vehicle. The more upset the patient is, the less able they become — which is true of all of us, with or without dementia. The best way — the only way — to deal with these "on" and "off" ability changes is with patience and understanding.

Of course, such symptoms occur with only some patients on the Alzheimer's spectrum. The vast majority shower, drive, and change clothes without difficulty until the end of their days. A patient of mine memorably played polo despite his dementia until he died in his late eighties of a gastrointestinal disorder.

SLEEP DISRUPTIONS

Sleep disruption is common in all of us as we age — older people have more trouble falling asleep, get fewer hours of sleep, and wake earlier. Compounding these issues, people with Alzheimer's may experience a disruption in their sleep-wake cycles and circadian rhythms, so that they tend to be up during the night and asleep during the day. (This disconnection between the internal and external clock can also occur in people without Alzheimer's, the die-hard "night owls.") About a quarter to a third of patients on the spectrum experience sleep changes. Prolonged inactivity during the day, which may be a consequence of dementia, also increases the tendency for daytime drowsiness and nighttime alertness. For this reason, I recommend that patients stay active during the day as much as possible.

Mavis was an 84-year-old widow with a full head of lustrous silver hair and a beautiful smile. The previous year, I had diagnosed her with slowly progressive Alzheimer's, with mild-moderate memory loss and good language and life skills. She was on medication and made her way to my office once a week to work on cognitive exercises with Casey, our superb psychologist. She was doing very well. A year into her treatment, we tested Mavis again and it appeared her Alzheimer's had stabilized.

A few months after those tests, I happened to be speaking to Mavis about the medications I was prescribing her when she casually mentioned that she took zolpidem (Ambien) nightly. I was stunned. This had never once come up before.

"Mavis! You're taking Ambien?"

"Yes," she said with a shrug. "Didn't I tell you about it?"

"No," I said. "Who gives it to you?"

It turned out that Mavis had been taking zolpidem nightly for nearly ten years. Her internist had first given her the prescription when her husband got sick. As his cancer progressed and she was taking care of him full time, she had stayed on it to ensure she was well rested. After his death, she continued to take it, and it had never occurred to her to tell me about it.

I told Mavis I thought it was best for her to stop taking the sleep aid, but she protested.

"It's only five milligrams," she objected. "I've been on it such a long time, and I'm doing well, aren't I?"

I agreed with her on all of her points, but I still thought there might be some cognitive benefits to her no longer taking zolpidem daily.

Mavis reluctantly agreed to try living without it, grumbling every step of the way. We slowly reduced her dose, so at the end of four months she was down to just a quarter pill daily. Then we tapered that down to every other day for a month. The following month, we got her down to a quarter pill every third day.

During the period of tapering and discontinuation of the zolpidem, Mavis's sleep was disrupted. I was not that concerned, because I knew the problem would ease over time as Mavis rid herself of both her physical and psychological dependence on the drug. Eventually, after Mavis had successfully been zolpidem-free for a month and a half, she told me that her sleep had returned to a normal pattern and she was no longer experiencing insomnia.

I was pleased to hear that, but the really pleasant surprise for both of us was the vast improvement in her memory once she stopped taking zolpidem. Suddenly, she was able to recite entire plots of movies, and, at one point, talked to me enthusiastically and in detail about all of the Academy Award picks for that year. This was a dramatic improvement, and I was astonished that such a small dose of zolpidem could have made such a big difference in her cognitive function. This experience made me believe even more firmly in the deleterious effects of sleeping medications like zolpidem in Alzheimer's disease.

I almost never prescribe medications like zolpidem (Ambien), zaleplon (Sonata), eszopiclone (Lunesta), and diazepam (Valium) for sleep in my practice, and I never do so for patients with Alzheimer's for two main reasons. First, larger doses are required over time for the drugs to keep working, which can make patients drowsy during the day. Second, these drugs interfere with a person's cognitive abilities by dulling their reflexes, much like alcohol does. My first line of treatment for patients with Alzheimer's who complain of sleep problems is melatonin, an over-the-counter sleep aid that helps to reset disrupted sleep cycles. If that fails, I try the herbal supplement valerian root, which is also available over the counter. If that also fails, I turn to prescription medications like trazodone, doxepin, and ramelteon, which are all helpful for sleep, are not addictive, and generally don't cause significant cognitive side effects.

IS IT APATHY OR IS IT DEPRESSION?
Apathy is a curious symptom, often seen in patients with dementia and just as often confused with depression. It is important to make the distinction between apathy and depression, because the treatment and prognosis for each is vastly different.

Harriet and her husband, Tom, were in my office because Harriet was convinced that 74-year-old Tom — who had slowly progressive Alzheimer's, with mild-moderate memory loss and good language and life skills — was depressed. In reality, he had an entirely different kind of problem.

"He's sitting around all day, completely disinterested. Our grandchildren came over the other day and he didn't even get off the couch," said Harriet, a quiet woman with short, blond hair who looked at me over wire-rimmed glasses. "I don't know what to do."

She was wearing a T-shirt that was too big for her, and I could see her clavicles where her shirt had fallen away from her neck. She had lost a lot of weight since Tom had received his diagnosis. All of her anxiety was laid bare in her increasingly scrawny neck.

Tom sat next to her, shaking his head. "I'm not depressed, Har," he protested. "I don't know what you mean. I'm not depressed at all."

"You sit there all day long, on the couch, watching television," she said, turning to face him. "Every single day! You don't want to do anything anymore! You don't want to go out with our friends; you don't want to play bridge. You used to play golf every Sunday, and you don't even do that now."

"That's because I want to watch the news," Tom replied calmly.

"Well, what was on the news yesterday?" Harriet asked, exasperated. "Can you tell me what was on the news yesterday?" All of a sudden, the meek Harriet had assumed the demeanor of a litigator at a trial.

"Well, it was the usual stuff," Tom said, shrugging.

"What usual stuff?" Harriet asked. "Just tell me — give me a couple of examples."

"I don't want to talk about it," Tom said. "It was, you know, the usual political stuff.

The stuff I like to watch."

"That's what I mean." Harriet sighed, turning back to me. "He has no idea what he's even been watching. Sometimes, I'll ask him to discuss what he's seen just a minute before on the screen and he can't tell me. I really do think he's not paying attention and is depressed."

Tom once again shook his head. "I'm not!" he exclaimed. "I'm really not."

I agreed with Tom. He wasn't depressed. He had apathy, a condition often mistaken for depression by caregivers. Because of the changes in the brain associated with Alzheimer's, the drive and initiative to start tasks or activities is often reduced. The patient will frequently not want to exercise, read, or go out to see friends, and almost certainly will not want to go to the doctor's office. Family members and caregivers often find this very trying and get into numerous arguments with the patient, like the one I had just witnessed between Tom and Harriet. They think they have to be the taskmasters, trying to get the patient to be more "active" and "involved" in day-to-day life.

"I have a whole list of things for Tom to do," Harriet told me. "I want him to get dressed and shave, I want him to go grocery shopping, but he won't do a thing. If he's not depressed, what is he?"

"Tom has something called apathy," I told her. "It's not depression. It's the result of a reduction in the drive that prompts most of us to do things. Although it might look like depression to you, Tom is perfectly content being, and not doing." I went on to explain that we can treat depression, but apathy is not treatable, although on occasion, stimulants like methylphenidate — Ritalin — may be of benefit.

"But isn't it important for his condition that he be more physically active?" Harriet asked. "Isn't it important that he stay mentally active, and socially active too? Isn't that what you've told us?"

"Yes, Harriet," I replied. "You're right. It is. And it's admirable that you're doing your best to make sure Tom is active. However, your role is not to be his therapist, his nurse, his scheduler, and his trainer. If you start to do all of those things, then you're not really going to be able to enjoy your most important role — that of being Tom's wife and partner."

I often counsel family members to have people around who are paid to fulfill at least some of the nonspouse roles, something that Medicare and Medicaid reimburse for in most states. If Tom was left to his own devices, he might never exercise. I told Harriet it was important to have somebody (not her!) come in and take Tom for a walk; it was also important to get one of his friends to come over to escort him to an occasional bridge game or a round of golf.

I also wanted Harriet to take care of herself. She recounted a visit from their son the previous week when he told her, "I don't understand why you are making such a fuss over Dad. He seems fine to me."

"I can't believe it," Harriet said, weeping in my office. "Does he even know how many times I have to listen to the same question? Does he know all the things I now have to do for Tom that he can't do himself? He thinks Tom is fine because Tom 'sounds reasonable,' but he isn't with Tom every hour of every day like I am."

This experience left Harriet feeling even lonelier and more isolated, a common experience for spouse caregivers. I suggested that she seek some professional mental health help, but she didn't think she needed it. I then advised Harriet to ask their son to spend a weekend with his father while she visited a friend or family member, or went to a spa. That would give her some much-needed respite and allow their son to appreciate how his father was doing and what his mother was going through. Although involving family and friends may put more of an onus on them, I sincerely believe it's an enriching experience for both the patient — because it extends their sense of community — and for the family members or friends who are stepping in. I, for one, find my admittedly limited alone time with my patients to be full of surprises, some delightful and some not, but always instructive and fulfilling. This is what I tried to convey to Harriet, but she believed in fighting a lonely war.

TREATING THE CAREGIVER

As we saw with Tom and Harriet, it may not just be the patient dealing with anxiety or depression or apathy. Quite often it is the caregiver who is affected. In fact, I believe Harriet was suffering more than Tom, who had become emotionally detached as the result of his illness. In Ben and Gail's case, Gail was the one who needed help for her anxiety.

Ben was a tall, suave, well-dressed man who had recently retired from running a multinational company. Over a period of forty years, he had worked his way up from being a stock boy to the CEO. By the time of his retirement, Ben had built up quite an empire.

When this savvy businessman found out at age 71 that he had slowly progressive Alzheimer's, he handled it with composure. "So I forget!" he would exclaim. "Everyone forgets! So I forget a little bit more than other people. What does it matter? It's not a big deal. It's not like I have cancer. I'm doing everything I can to treat this — that's the best I can do."

His wife, Gail, meanwhile, was devastated by her husband's diagnosis. She was a nervous wreck to the point that she eventually needed to go on antidepressants to calm down.

Ben warned me early on, "Don't you pay attention to my wife. She's a nervous Nellie, and this has thrown her for a loop."

Every time Ben forgot something, no matter how insignificant, Gail called me. "He forgot to take his keys," she would say. "He wanted to wear the same pair of trousers two days in a row." Every day, there was something else. "He didn't know which exit to get off when he was driving. Does this mean he's getting worse? Does this mean he's going to die next year? Does this mean he's about to lose his mind?"

Sometimes, this would happen in my office when both of them were present. Ben would turn to her and say, "Can you cut that out already? Relax!" But his wife simply wasn't able to.

Gail understood she was a worrywart and that her anxiety served no constructive purpose, yet she was simply unable to stop. Once, in absolute exasperation, I said to her jokingly, "I am going to lock you in the closet and throw away the key!"

"Not a bad idea," she said, laughing. We had reached a stage where she would let me gently tease her about her anxiety. "I know I can get pretty nuts sometimes."

I got a call from her internist the very next day. "Gayatri," he said, "I heard you threatened to lock up Gail yesterday. I wish I'd thought of that years ago. She is a sweetheart, but boy, does she work herself up into a tizzy."

The charm of Gail was that she had a sense of humor about her anxiety. She didn't take what I said as an affront, but rather as a sign of my own frustration at being unable to calm her down.

After much cajoling, her internist and I persuaded Gail to see a psychiatrist, who prescribed an antidepressant that also helped her anxiety. Ben was very pleased with the results.

"She's a lot easier to live with now," Ben told me. "We should have done this forty years ago. If only I had known!"

It is important to attend to the emotional needs of both patients and their caregivers. Their needs are intertwined. The mental health of each affects the other to a larger degree than in relationships where neither partner is on the spectrum. The good news is that anxiety and depression can be successfully treated, improving quality of life for both.

CHAPTER 9
I'D BE CRAZY NOT TO BE PARANOID!
APRAXIA, PARANOIA, AND OTHER FRUSTRATING BEHAVIORS, AND HOW TO EFFECTIVELY COMMUNICATE WHEN LOGIC DOESN'T WORK

Some patients on the severe end of the Alzheimer's spectrum develop behaviors that can puzzle and frustrate caregivers and family members. A trusting father may suddenly accuse his children of stealing from him; a cooperative husband may apply toothpaste to a comb or refuse to let go of the car door; a reasonable parent may insist that a stranger is coming into the home and rearranging things. These behaviors are not borne out of a patient's desire to annoy their caregivers or seek attention, but are caused by brain-related difficulties with translating ideas into action. To deal with these issues effectively, one must understand the reasons behind them. This will not only alleviate a caregiver's bewilderment and anxiety, but also help the patient feel more understood and, consequently, less agitated.

THE INS AND OUTS OF APRAXIA

"He is fine when it's a relaxing day," Cora, the wife of my patient Junior, told me. "But on days when I'm in a hurry, trying to get out the door to work, Junior can't seem to do a thing by himself. Not even put on his trousers! It's like he's doing it on purpose to aggravate me, to try to get me to stay home with him. The other day I asked him to brush his teeth, and he was in the bathroom a long time. I finally checked, and he had the toothpaste squeezed out all over the sink instead of on his brush. I couldn't help myself: I yelled, 'Junior, what are you doing?' Since I yelled at him, he has had no problems brushing his teeth. It seems to me that he was doing it on purpose. This man has enjoyed aggravating me his whole life!"

I told Cora, who was still working part-time as a travel agent, that it sounded to me like her husband was suffering from apraxia: an inability to perform a previously learned task like dressing or making coffee. I explained that even though it felt as if yelling at Junior was a good solution, it was not. It was becoming hard for Junior to translate a mental idea like getting dressed into a sequence of actions for himself: first underclothes, then socks, then shirt, then pants, then belt, then shoes. He might put on his underwear over his pants, or omit his pants, or wear just his shirt. This might happen some days but not others. The brain circuits for doing such automatic, sequenced actions sometimes worked for Junior but not always, just like a faulty light switch sometimes turns on the bulb, but at other times doesn't. Medication does not help with apraxia, but understanding and responding to the symptoms of the condition behaviorally can be effective in dealing with the problem.

Ideomotor — translating a mental idea into a motor act — apraxia can occur with actions that all of us were taught to perform as children and now do almost automatically. Apraxia may be the culprit when patients try to answer the phone when the doorbell rings and when they don't change out of clothes they've been wearing for a week. Other commonly affected sequences include putting on makeup, using the toilet, taking a shower, and eating. Because these are daily activities, caregivers like Cora can be particularly frustrated when mental switches for them fail. To her, it felt like it was a voluntary choice on her husband's part to suddenly become inept, especially when she was in a hurry. Adding an element of urgency to a motor act makes us all more prone to panic and poorer performance. We all make more mistakes when we are being hurried, whether we fall on the Alzheimer's spectrum or not.

The good news is that most patients never develop apraxia, or have only a mild version of it. And patients who do have apraxia, like Junior, can still function well in other areas. He enjoyed talking with me at great length about airplane engines, his hobby. Once I explained apraxia to Cora and made it clear that Junior was not failing on purpose, she was able to handle his episodes much more easily. She realized that he was apraxic with certain things, like dressing and grooming, but not with eating, washing the dishes, or folding clothes. So, she helped him dress, and he helped her clean around the house.

"I finally got myself a housekeeping helper," she said when we next met, "even though I have to help him brush his teeth." Cora was much more relaxed this time around.

TROUBLE SWALLOWING

Holly was a tiny woman in her eighties with Alzheimer's and a penchant for wearing brightly patterned tights — even as her dementia advanced. Because of her apraxia, she was not able to feed herself well. She could no longer use utensils appropriately, for example, and would try to cut meat with a spoon. Her husband was concerned because she was losing weight, so he would try to feed her.

"The problem is that she won't swallow," he told me. "She keeps food in the side of her mouth, and sometimes, when I finally look, almost her entire breakfast is stored in her cheeks." Holly did not spit out her food — another motor action — but instead stored it inside her cheeks, trying to please her husband, whom she sensed wanted her to eat.

Holly's brain was having difficulty activating the mechanism for the swallowing process. I told Holly's husband to check to make sure she wasn't storing food in her cheeks between mouthfuls. An easy way to help make sure food is being swallowed is to give the patient sips of fluid between each bite, as the swallowing of fluid is more automatic than the swallowing of solids and helps to wash everything down. Thankfully, this didn't happen every time Holly ate; there were meals when her brain's swallowing switch worked fine.

TROUBLE SITTING DOWN

Another symptom of dementia that can be hard for caregivers to understand is a patient's difficulty with coordinating their bodies spatially within their environment. Loss of the sense of where the body is in space can result in patients sitting on the edge of a chair seat, or on the arm, or missing the chair entirely. They may reach for a glass of water and miss it completely or reach past it and spill it in the process. They may place a cup of coffee in midair instead of on a table. Infants and toddlers do this as well, but they learn to be more coordinated as they grow older. As with other kinds of apraxia, medications are of little help here — it's better to do your best to modify the environment to avoid potential hazards. Help patients navigate directly into their chairs, use covered containers — and just be prepared for spills!

NOT KNOWING

Agnosia is a condition whereby a patient loses the concept of what something is or how it is to be used. In extreme cases, when

I give a patient a pen, for instance, she may not only hold it awkwardly, but also may not know its name or its function. A patient may not know what a comb is, and also not know how to hold or use it. A remote control may be used to try to ladle soup. A doorknob may lose its meaning as the mechanism to get past a shut door.

A memorable example of agnosia occurred early in my career with an elegant woman who wore beautiful silk dresses and, even in her nineties, carried around a little black, ostrich-skin handbag. At one point her caregiver discovered, with not a small amount of horror, that my patient was storing pieces of her feces in her beloved purse.

She would insist on taking her handbag with her into the bathroom, but instead of flushing the toilet after a bowel movement, she removed well-formed sections of feces and placed them in her handbag. She refused to part with her feces because she believed it was precious. Children are not born with a natural aversion to handling feces, but they develop it. Unfortunately, my patient had lost this aversion as the result of her dementia and developed an agnosia for feces. This was a memorable example, but thankfully, one that doesn't happen very often. Agnosia is not responsive to medication, but behavioral solutions sometimes work. In this particular situation, for instance, we were eventually able to coax my patient into leaving her handbag behind when using the bathroom.

LOGIC HAS NOTHING TO DO WITH IT

Another symptom that can arise in some men and women with dementia is called *gegenhalten* — which, in the German translation, means "counterpressure." Anyone who has spent any time with babies knows that you can hold out two fingers and they will latch on with their little hands so tightly that you can pick them up that way. Their grasp reflex is instinctive — they can't choose to not grasp or to let go. As we grow, we are able to override this reflex — we grasp only when we want and let go when we want. This ability to override the grasp reflex of infancy is lost in some patients on the spectrum and is one of the most common examples of *gegenhalten*. Resistance to other passive movements, such as when a caregiver is trying to get a patient out of a chair, can occur. Milly and Walt exemplify some of the common issues related to *gegenhalten*.

"Walt is perfectly fine when he wants to be," his wife, Milly, told me. "But the other day, I was trying to move him out of his armchair and into bed, and he began clinging to the chair. The more I tried to get him to move, the harder he held on. I ended up screaming, 'Walt! Let go! Let go!' but he wouldn't do it. Finally, I walked away and came back awhile later. He then got up from the chair and into bed without problems."

I explained to Milly that Walt was experiencing *gegenhalten.* Walt was 84 and had been diagnosed four years earlier with slowly progressive Alzheimer's with mild memory, language, and life skills problems. The switch in Walt's brain that let him override his primal grasp reflex was malfunctioning. His hands grasped his chair with the same intensity as the infant Walt might have used to cling to his mother's fingers when she swung him playfully in the air over his crib 83 years ago. Milly had instinctively done the right thing — she had walked away and come back a few minutes later, at which point the reflex action was not switched on.

I asked Milly whether Walt grasped on to other things, and she replied, "He sometimes has trouble letting go of the car-door handle when we go places. And on occasion he holds on to his fork as if it were glued to his palm."

Walt was also having difficulties with

flushing the toilet, partly because of *gegen-halten* — he couldn't let the tank handle go — and partly as the result of apraxia (he'd lost the ability to complete a sequential motor act — using and then flushing the toilet).

"Walt believes the toilet is broken," Milly said. "It happens to be a great toilet and works instantly with one flush. He now has this habit of pulling and holding the handle down without releasing it, which results in the tank not filling up. Walt wants to call a plumber, even though I show him that when I flush it, it works perfectly."

"Milly," I said, "how are *you* doing?"

"I'm okay," she said. "Ninety percent of the time, I am doing really well. But when Walt gets angry and yells, it gets me upset."

"Does he get most upset with you when you show him what he is doing wrong?" I asked.

She told me yes.

"Well, this may sound odd, but I suggest that rather than showing him that he is not flushing correctly, agree with him that there is a problem with the toilet. He is happy thinking that there is something wrong with the toilet's flushing mechanism and not with his brain. Let him. His rationalizations give him dignity and help him save face. Pointing out his error is not going to help. I know you are all for honesty, but I believe the best thing to do here is agree with him. When you don't, what he hears is 'You are so stupid, you don't even know how to flush the toilet.' "

"But that's not very logical," she said.

"Logic has nothing to do with it," I replied. "When you try to communicate logically in these circumstances, both you and Walt will end up frustrated and angry."

Once Milly understood the cause of Walt's actions, it was easier for her to both deal with it and to be more empathic with her husband. Walt couldn't let go even if he wanted to. He was at times, quite literally, stuck.

I find it effective to both support the caregiver's feelings and explain the underlying process so that the behavior, inexplicable though it seems, makes neurologic sense. Thorough explanations and advice about dealing with symptoms like *gegenhalten* and apraxia lead to better communication between the caregiver and the patient and reduce caregiver stress.

SHH . . . SHE'S LISTENING: PARANOIA

"Where is she? Can she hear us?" one of my favorite patients Mo asked me in hushed tones. We were at the beginning of our cognitive exercises, and he was sitting across from me, leaning in.

I asked Mo what he meant, and he repeated himself. "Where is she?" he whispered. "Can you hear her?"

"Who are you talking about?" I asked, perplexed.

"Martha," Mo whispered conspiratorially.

"Your wife?" I asked.

"Yes," he mouthed at me. "Where is she?"

"I think she's gone out for a cup of coffee and to take a walk," I told Mo. "That's usually what she does when we're doing these exercises. She is not in the office, and she can't hear us."

"Well," he said, "she's been hitting me." He looked at me sadly through his glasses, his appealing face suffused with woe.

This came as an enormous shock, because Mo's wife, Martha, was one of the most devoted caregivers I had ever met — she adored her husband. A former middle school teacher, she oozed a firm kindness that only someone who'd spent decades guiding squirmy preteens could. Martha listened to Mo struggle to remember events and finish phrases with a level of patience that I found remarkable. I had never observed her even interrupting her husband, yet here she was being accused of physical assault. I was dumbfounded.

"What do you mean, she's been hitting you?" I asked.

"When we get into bed, she pushes me to the side," Mo said, "away from her."

I said nothing, relieved that Mo was misinterpreting a relatively simple gesture as something more serious.

Then he said, "She's been seeing someone."

"Who?" I asked.

"My friend Joe," Mo told me earnestly. "I've known Joe since high school, and his wife died two years ago. Martha told me before we got married that she had a crush on him. And now I see them together all the time."

When I first met Mo nearly seven years earlier, he was a shell of his former self. He had found out inadvertently that he had Alzheimer's, after calling his internist's office to find out the results of an MRI that had been ordered for his memory complaints. The secretary on the end of the line had told him bluntly, "The scan says it looks like you have Alzheimer's disease. You have some brain shrinkage."

Mo was devastated, because this condition was something he had dreaded. Both of his parents had died from Alzheimer's.

He told me later, "I hung up the phone and felt like I had hung up on my life."

He was 68 when he heard this news, and although he had already retired from his business a few years previously, he had spent his days outside, socializing with his buddies and golfing. After the telephone call, he began to stay home, frightened for his future and depressed. When Martha urged him to see the doctor even just to find out if the receptionist was accurate in her reporting on Mo's scan, he refused, telling Martha, "I knew it all along. It was only a matter of time."

Mo became my patient early in my career, and we took to each other quickly, becoming co-combatants in the battle against his illness. I diagnosed him at age 70 with slowly progressive Alzheimer's disease with mild memory loss and intact language and life skills. In addition to treating him with medication, I met with Mo for weekly brain exercises, running through a multitude of exercises to keep his brain as active as possible. During this time, we developed a close relationship.

Slowly, Mo came out of his shell and became much more engaged. He played with his grandchildren again, and Mo and Martha even started to take vacations.

The story of Martha's affair came as a surprise to me. Mo was convincing in his low-key relating of the story, and despite my high index of suspicion for paranoia in patients with Alzheimer's, as well as my background in psychiatry and neurology, I was taken in. I could understand how it could have happened. After all, Mo spoke with assurance, and Martha was a very good-looking woman, who wore beautifully tailored suits that showed her legs off to advantage. She seemed a likely candidate for the first female caregiver to have an affair in my practice.

As I listened to Mo's story, with its vivid details and his clear distress, I slowly became upset on his behalf. I wondered why Martha couldn't have chosen someone further afield. But I counseled Mo to wait a little while and see how things played out.

Mo and Martha remained on my mind for days. When Mo came in for his session the following week, there was even more to the story.

"Martha's been stealing my money," he said. "She took money from my wallet. She's been taking money from our bank account and siphoning it into her own account. She's doing it because they are going to run away together. Martha and Joe are going to run away and get married and leave me alone."

It was at that point that I realized that Mo had become paranoid. His tales had been just that — tales, fiction — but I had been taken in. This was partly because I harbored a deep fondness for Mo and clucked over his progress in the manner of a proud mother hen. But it was also because Mo spoke with a conviction that was very persuasive. It can be difficult to recognize paranoia in a patient, even for an expert.

I recall many instances where family members have fought with one another based on a patient's paranoid accusations, believing them to be true. As it did for Mo, paranoia in Alzheimer's often centers, like a Greek tragedy, on fidelity and finances, which can cause familial strife when the paranoia is not recognized for what it is.

Once I finally recognized that Mo was paranoid, I prescribed a small dose of the antipsychotic medication olanzapine, and his symptoms cleared up in just two weeks. He went back to trusting his wife and quickly forgot his paranoid episode. Mo was stable for three more years before his dementia began to progress further and he died, still recognizing his beloved Martha.

Paranoia generally develops later in the

course of Alzheimer's as the brain works overtime to make sense of the chronic forgetfulness that accompanies dementia, although sometimes it can be the earliest symptom. Patients can be convinced that someone came into their home and stole from them, or that the people who are closest to them are playing cruel tricks on them. When patients start forgetting things, it can be easier for them to accept the idea that there is a conspiracy against them than it is to accept that they are losing their mind.

Bearing the brunt of a paranoid patient's accusations is difficult for caregivers and family. It helps if they understand the neurologic reasons for the unfounded accusations.

THE ROOTS OF PARANOIA

Elena was a 78-year-old patient with slowly progressive Alzheimer's, with mild-moderate memory loss and excellent language and life skills. Although she had no trouble driving, she struggled daily to remember where she had parked her car. She would be utterly convinced it was in one location, when she'd actually left it in another. Her loving husband of fifty-two years, Sal, regularly had to tell her that she was wrong and prove it to her by taking her to the correct location.

This was so confusing and disorienting for Elena that she became convinced that Sal was moving the car without telling her, just to make her look bad.

Her suspicions grew as her condition worsened. One morning, Elena was positive that she had put her glasses down next to her newspaper on the kitchen table while she and Sal were having breakfast. When she returned from the bathroom to find neither newspaper nor glasses on the table, she was sure Sal had something to do with it, particularly as he'd been sitting right there the whole time.

"Where did you put my glasses and the paper?" she asked, annoyed.

"I didn't touch them," Sal said, continuing to munch nonchalantly on his bacon and eggs. "I think you took them with you when you got up."

Elena was indignant at the suggestion. "Now, why would I do that?" she snapped.

Sure enough, though, Sal was correct; Elena had left both on the hall table on her way to the bathroom.

This type of thing began to occur on a daily basis for Elena. Every time something went missing, Sal magically seemed to know where it was. As the number of these confusing incidents mounted, Elena's suspicions of her husband grew steadily. She began to accuse him of playing tricks on her.

"I have no idea what to do," Sal said. "I can't seem to do anything right. I am always the bad guy." He was at his wits' end, sad, angry, and frustrated.

RESPONDING TO THE UNSPOKEN MESSAGE

Being a full-time caregiver of a person with Alzheimer's disease is a 24-hour-a-day, 7-day-a-week, 365-day-a-year task, with no breaks, no recognition, and no light at the end of the tunnel. It is an extremely tough job and not for the faint of heart. Family caregivers are handed the job without any training, and for many, it is the toughest job of their lives.

For people who are already living in these exhausting and upsetting conditions, feeling trapped and helpless, it can cause even more anger to be falsely accused by the person who is their unwitting prisoner in this emotionally and physically depleting role.

Caregivers are faced with these challenges on a daily basis, and when they take it personally (and it's hard not to), even the smallest of hurdles can sometimes feel insurmountable. It is essential for caregivers who are dealing with false accusations to stay mindful that these charges are not a reflection on them. Rather they are reflective of the patient's struggle to maintain some semblance of control over their deteriorating world.

The easiest way to tackle this issue is to avoid confrontation as much as possible. How? In Elena and Sal's case, we discovered that the quickest way to handle Elena's confusion about where the car was parked was for Sal to own up to something he didn't do. This was as simple as him saying, "You know what, honey? I moved the car and completely forgot to tell you about it. I apologize for that." You might think that having Elena write down where her car was parked or snap a cell phone photo showing its location would work, but in my experience, these tricks don't. It's not likely that Elena would remember to create the reminder in the first place, and even if she did, she'd likely forget to check it or have misplaced it when the time came.

Handling Elena's forgetfulness in this gentle way made her feel vindicated and helped her retain her sense of dignity. By telling these white lies, Sal avoided an argument and enabled them to carry on with their day, free of stress and drama.

If Sal had insisted on clinging to the facts,

it would have caused countless arguments, as well as a great deal of angst for Elena. For her, this wasn't about the car, it was a direct personal attack on the integrity of her brain, and she would fight fiercely to maintain her dignity. This is why I tell families of patients with Alzheimer's, "Don't fight the little things."

BEING MISLEADING OR BEING SUPPORTIVE?

Some caregivers find such an approach repugnant: the "lying" to a patient, or colluding with the delusion. Others may think that it's pandering or patronizing to them. I see it as simply assuaging a patient's underlying fears, without forcing them to face the fact that they have lost their grip on reality and are being paranoid. I see it as replying to the patient's unspoken question, "Have I lost my mind?" with the caregiver's unspoken answer, "No, you have not; I'm the one who made a mistake."

To make this approach more palatable, we must keep in mind that regardless of whether or not we fall on the Alzheimer's spectrum, our brains are evolutionarily geared to fight back against any perceived attack on our competence. For example, I park my car on the streets of New York City every day, and like Elena, I often forget where it is. Sometimes, I am entirely convinced I parked it in a specific spot, and when my car is not there, rather than questioning my belief, I assume it has been towed or stolen. To instinctively blame the external environment rather than one's own strong conviction is the default mode for all our brains. This is ultimately the root of the paranoia in patients on the Alzheimer's spectrum.

Trying to explain reality to the patient (or me) is not going to help. It serves only to make the patient (or me) feel less competent and capable. Going along with what a patient believes, even when it feels utterly preposterous, is ultimately the kinder thing to do.

CORRECTING OR ACCEPTING A FALSE BELIEF

Estie, the daughter of one of my patients, told me, "Dad keeps saying he's going to work every morning. Should I allow him to think this? Or should I keep doing what I've been doing, which is to correct him and say, 'No, Dad. You retired from your job years ago. You haven't gone to work in more than a decade. Don't you remember?'

"Of course, he doesn't remember," she

continued. "We have to go through the whole thing again, every day: the retirement party, the gold pen that he got as a gift, which I then show him and which he doesn't recognize. Then we go through it all again the next day — or even worse, an hour later. On bad days, fifteen minutes later. I feel if I don't correct him, then I'm helping his dementia progress," she concluded, expressing a concern I hear frequently from caregivers. "Is this the case?"

"No," I reassured Estie. "It's not. This is not neurologically or neuroscientifically possible."

I believe that effective communication with a patient with dementia means supporting their brain's ability to organize the world as they see it, in a manner that doesn't affront their dignity, while still allowing them to function. I instruct families to collude with whatever belief system a patient has, unless it's something that is clearly going to be harmful to them. For example, if a patient insists on getting dressed and going out to work in the middle of the night, rather than tell them that they don't work anymore and it's the middle of the night, redirect them into the bedroom and say, "Today is a holiday." To phrase it in terms that might make sense, without harming their pride, is the best way to cope with the issue.

I cannot recall a single instance in my years of practice when correcting a patient's firmly held belief was urgent, important, or actually led to a consistent change in his or her belief system. Even if they agree in the moment, soon enough patients revert to the more strongly held preexisting belief, such as the one that says it's time for work or the car is in Section B of the lot. The given correction is often forgotten quickly and creates only agitation. My general opinion in these situations is to allow the patient the dignity of maintaining a semblance of self-knowledge, regardless of whether it is valid.

DENYING ILLNESS

Sometimes patients don't believe there's anything wrong with them and deny their illness because of a deficit in their self-awareness. This condition is called anosognosia, and can occur as a result of certain types of strokes and psychiatric conditions; it can also manifest with some patients on the Alzheimer's spectrum.

My patient Adam was a good example of this. At 78, he was balding, wore glasses, and had a thousand-watt smile. Adam proffered quick and witty answers to my questions.

"What brings you here?" I asked at the start of our first meeting.

"I don't remember," he said, laughing.

His wife, sitting next to him, shook her head and scolded, "Adam, be serious!"

Adam looked at her with a flash of anger. "I am serious!" he exclaimed. "Isn't that what you've been telling me? That I can't remember and I need to be here?"

His wife turned to me helplessly.

"Adam doesn't believe he has a problem," she said. "He doesn't think there's anything wrong with his memory. But he keeps repeating himself, and the other day he forgot that it was our son's birthday — and he's never forgotten something like that before."

"I knew it was our son's birthday all along," Adam protested. "I wanted to see if *she'd* remember."

"Adam," his wife replied, "that's simply not true. All right, then, tell me his date of birth."

"His date of birth?" Adam replied. "Ha ha. His date of birth is the day he was born. Anyone could answer that!"

"You see what I mean," his wife said, turning back to me. "He has no idea when our son was born."

This was a classic back-and-forth that occurs when patients deny they have memory problems, and caregivers keep insisting that they do.

I turned to Adam. "It's clear that you're here under protest," I said. "And I'm sorry that you're feeling this way. Let's try to get this over with quickly so you can be on your way."

Adam agreed, and after a while he began to thaw.

"How do you think your mind is?" I asked. "Do you think it's working the way it always has?"

"It's slowed down a little bit," Adam confessed. "I can't seem to remember things the way that I used to. But my poker buddies all tell me my memory is better than theirs. Forgetting is a normal sign of aging, isn't it?"

In his question, I heard concern and not a small amount of fear. I sensed that Adam was worried about losing his memory, but he wasn't yet ready to deal with it. So I went along with him.

"It can be," I told him. "We're going to have to do some tests to figure out if your memory problem is simply related to you getting older or something else is going on.

The earlier we intervene, the more success-ful we'll be in taking care of the problem."

Adam's approach — outwardly denying his memory loss while still nursing niggling doubts — is common. Some patients com-pletely deny memory loss, and others, after the diagnosis is made, deny the results. Adam did a little of each. He was found to have Alzheimer's but never accepted it, and aside from rare instances, denied having memory problems. Faced with a situation like this, the caregiver may insist on repeat-edly telling the patient that they have Alz-heimer's. Some of them will bring out troves of evidence to support their contention, such as medications, appointments missed, items misplaced, and things repeated, but the patient usually has a counterargument to everything.

"You forgot your glasses," the caregiver might say.

"They weren't working well for me any-way," the patient will say. "I need a new set."

"You forgot your keys," the caregiver might say.

"Well, why do I need keys?" the patient will protest. "You have them in your hand-bag! Why would I need to bring them along as well?"

Or: "Do you remember how many years

we have been married?"

The patient doesn't know, so she may counter with "Long enough to have known better!" or, "Too long!" or "Why don't *you* tell *me*?"

A common problem for caregivers is getting the patient in for a memory evaluation in the first place. Many patients are reluctant, and some outright refuse.

"There's nothing wrong with my memory. I'm not crazy," a husband might say to his wife. "Why don't you get *your* memory checked?"

I counsel family members to tell loved ones that they are being taken in for a neurologic evaluation — this is in fact more accurate than to call it a memory evaluation and also feels less threatening. I also recommend that the family say that the reason for the evaluation is to allow the patient to keep their brain healthy and allow them to stay independent as they get older. This is vastly different from telling someone that they need to have their memory evaluated because they might be getting Alzheimer's. Numerous surveys have revealed that the threat of Alzheimer's is the deepest fear of people over the age of 65, more dreaded than a cancer diagnosis. The threat of the loss of independence is scarier to us than the prospect of death. The patient needs to be told that the evaluation is a step toward independence, not nursing home placement, as is usually feared.

Some patients don't like to be reminded of the possibility of Alzheimer's because they remember someone on the severe end of the spectrum and don't want to have a similar label applied to them. Some worry about what the future holds for them and prefer to deny rather than get distraught when conjuring up this future.

Effective Communication in Alzheimer's

Some things to consider to facilitate communication in patients with dementia:

- Paranoia is a method of self-defense in Alzheimer's that allows the person to cope with memory loss without acknowledging the severity of cognitive loss.
- In responding to patients, it's more important to be emotionally correct than it is to be factually correct.
- It's okay if a patient denies memory loss, so long as they comply with treatment.
- Violence on the part of someone with Alzheimer's disease almost always stems from a perceived threat to personal safety, rather than from intent to do harm.
- In situations where there is paranoia or

the potential for violence, redirection is more effective and more dignity-preserving than confrontation.

NONDIRECTED VIOLENCE

Patients with Alzheimer's may lash out when they are forced to do something that makes them anxious, even if it's a mundane activity like taking a shower. Such violence is almost always nondirected — in other words, it's aimed not at hurting someone, but rather at avoiding a perceived harm. For example, when a patient pushes away a caregiver who is trying to get them into the bathtub, the patient's aim is not to hurt the caregiver but to prevent the caregiver from hurting them by putting them into the bathtub, which may be something the patient is afraid of. In other words, the violence often stems from patient anxiety, lack of comprehension, and fear, rather than malice toward another.

"It's been the worst week of my life," Alan, my patient Josie's husband, told me.

"What happened?" I asked.

"It's Josie," he said, gesturing to his wife of forty-five years. "Yesterday, she got into bed with me and asked who I was. 'What do you mean?' I said. 'I'm Alan! Your husband!' At first I thought she was joking, but then I realized from the look in her eyes that she was scared. 'I'm Alan! Alan! Your husband!' I insisted. And you know what she said? 'You're not Alan. You're too old to be Alan. Who is Alan anyway? Where's Dad?' It was like this throughout the night. Sometimes she knew me, and at other times, she said she was waiting for her parents to come home.

"I tried telling her all about our lives," Alan continued. "I told her she was Josie, that we've been married for forty-five years, that we have children together. She seemed to understand, and then at other times she was confused. At one point, she tried to push me off the bed because she got so angry and upset with me."

Violence of this type is deeply disturbing to caregivers, as is, of course, not being recognized by a spouse of many decades, and it's frightening for both parties concerned. There was no way to get Josie to recognize Alan in the moment. Time needed to elapse, and the bedroom light had to be turned on to increase orientation cues to calm Josie down. Bringing out the wedding albums and the photos of the children was not going to help. Josie needed to feel understood; she was scared and confused.

Understanding the motivation for the

patient's aggression is helpful. Behavioral interventions, aimed at the underlying cause — such as apraxia — rather than the actual act — toothpaste on the comb — is helpful. Almost always, however, treatment with medication is also necessary. Various types of medication, including antidepressants and antipsychotics, are effective in treating violence and frequently eliminate it because they reduce the underlying anxiety that leads to such behavior.

By effectively intuiting and perceiving a patient's needs, the lives of both patients and caregivers can be immeasurably improved. Whether the issue is one of false accusations of stolen money or of food sequestered in the mouth, the cause is neurological and not personal. The response should therefore be directed toward supporting and treating the brain disorder with behavioral and environmental modifications, as well as medications when indicated.

CHAPTER 10
I'M NOT LOST — I'M ON THE ROAD LESS TRAVELED. WHY NOT TO WORRY ABOUT WANDERING

One of the biggest fears for caregivers of patients with Alzheimer's is that the patient will get lost and harm will befall them. Caregivers can find themselves in the stressful position of constraining the movements of their fiercely independent loved ones, and patients can feel unnecessarily controlled by their caregivers and resent it. One of my patients began to fight with his loving and concerned wife, referring to her as a "spoilsport" and other, even less flattering terms, which often reduced her to helpless tears. I try to address caregiver concerns by reassuring them that, in my experience, lost patients are eventually located, and they're usually safe and sound.

In twenty-three years of practice dealing with hundreds of patients across the Alzheimer's spectrum, only seven have gotten lost, and all were found within twenty-four hours. Five eventually found their way home, sometimes by asking for help, and two were found after a relatively quick search. One person got lost while driving and finally pulled into a gas station a few hundred miles from home and asked for assistance. The others got lost on foot. Although there are exceptions to the rule, I have found that even when patients are wandering the streets at night in their pajamas, it's rare for significant harm to befall them.

A MOVIE OR THE OPERA?

You might recall Dr. Samuels, the psychoanalyst in Chapter 4 who continued to practice successfully despite his failing memory. I remember one occasion when his wife, Doris, called me, frantic because he had gone missing. She had come home from the movies to discover he wasn't home. They'd had an argument at the movie theater earlier that evening over the fact that he had wanted to go to the opera but she had wanted to see a film. Dr. Samuels stomped off in the middle of this squabble, and his wife watched as he got into a cab and headed home — or so she thought.

When she returned home at 10:00 p.m. and discovered he wasn't there, she panicked and called me. I did my best to reassure her, telling her that patients with Alzheimer's usually find their way home, with or without help, and suggested she sit tight for a little while.

Despite my counsel, Doris called the police. She told me later that when the police arrived, they conducted a thorough search of the apartment, including inside closets, as Doris watched in bewilderment. "What were they looking for there?" she asked.

After this futile search, the police told her that they could not file a missing person's report, not only because Dr. Samuels was an adult and had been missing for less than twenty-four hours, but because they didn't believe that a practicing physician could have Alzheimer's disease. This happened years ago, before most states introduced the Silver Alert law, which allows caregivers to notify the authorities about missing adults with dementia well before twenty-four hours are up.

Dr. Samuels eventually showed up at about 11:30 that evening. He strolled casually into the apartment with a big smile on his face. Turns out, he had decided to go to the opera after all and found a single center orchestra seat, from which he enjoyed Puccini's *Aida*. He was rather pleased with himself and couldn't understand what all the fuss was about, having completely forgotten their earlier argument.

NOT ALL WHO WANDER ARE LOST

Another patient who got "lost" was Giuliana, an immigrant from Sicily. One crisp fall day, Giuliana's daughter, Stephanie, arrived at my office with her mother and her two children in tow. Stephanie lived two blocks away from her mother on Staten Island and was very concerned about Giuliana's worsening memory.

"I don't know what's the matter with my daughter," Giuliana exclaimed as she sat opposite me after my initial examination. "There's nothing wrong with me. She says there's a problem with my mind, *capisce*? I'm fine! My husband says I'm fine. Doctor, look at me! I'm fine, yes?"

I suspected Giuliana was suffering from a form of dementia, most likely Alzheimer's. She showed several telltale signs. She had a large handbag with many unusual things in it, and as she dived into it to retrieve her medications, I noticed gardening gloves and a small drinking glass. She had three different wallets, one with her credit cards in it, another with her driver's license and other cards, and yet another with more cards and her medication list, along with multiple bits of paper on which she had scribbled reminders to herself. Such overstuffed bags are often signs of memory dysfunction. I have sometimes found passports and multiple copies of unpaid and unopened bills in the bags of my patients with dementia. Patients carry with them important pieces of information that they are worried they will forget or misplace. Of course, because this was the first time I had met Giuliana, she needed testing to confirm my preliminary impression.

Meanwhile, Giuliana's daughter, Stephanie, waited patiently outside in the reception room, tending to her toddler son and her infant daughter. In an effort to keep the two youngsters amused, she decided to take them out for a walk until my meeting with Giuliana was over. As the three of them left, she informed my receptionist where she would be and let her know she wouldn't be long.

Unfortunately, when Stephanie came back to get her mother at five o'clock, Giuliana had vanished. Somehow in the blink of an eye, she had managed to escape the waiting room and gone out into the alien landscape of New York City. To make matters worse, she had left the office without her coat that

October evening. Giuliana had lived in Staten Island all of her American life. Remarkably, until that day she had not once stepped foot in Manhattan, despite her proximity to it. She told me that she had been completely satisfied running a small grocery store in her neighborhood and never felt the urge to visit the Big Apple.

As you can imagine, we were all dismayed about Giuliana's disappearance. Although I was inwardly a little panicked, I remained calm. Stephanie, on the other hand, broke down crying immediately.

"My mother has never been in Manhattan before," she said, sobbing. "She's afraid of the city. She always said, 'Too many cars! Too many people!' And now I've brought her here and she's lost."

Noticing his mother's distress, Stephanie's toddler burst into tears as well, and the office was quickly plunged into a state of bedlam. I tried to maintain a cool demeanor.

"I know we'll find your mother, Stephanie," I said. "I'm sure she's not far away. It's true that she has her wallet with her, but I doubt she'll go anywhere without you. She doesn't know how to hail a cab, much less use the subway."

Given the late hour of the day, I decided

to close the office a little early and have my staff spread out on foot to look for Giuliana. I knew there was no point in calling the police to assist — Giuliana had been gone less than half an hour, not nearly long enough to rise to the top of the priority list.

Joining me on this frantic search was my daughter, Ginny, who was ten years old at the time. She had happened to be dropped off from school just as we realized Giuliana was missing. "Mom, what's the matter?" she asked.

"We have to go and look for a lost patient," I told her. To her credit, this answer didn't faze her one bit and she was ready to pitch in.

I plotted out the routes we would each take, feeling rather like an army general. "You take Lexington, then Third Avenue," I told my secretary. "Go up and down the avenues — don't take the side streets."

I sent our psychologist to Madison Avenue, and my nurse, an independent thinker, decided to go in whatever direction her intuition took her. Meanwhile, Ginny and I decided to search Park Avenue with my dogs, whom I brought with me to work daily. I asked Stephanie to crisscross the side streets and to leave her cell phone on.

As we roamed Park Avenue, five o'clock

turned to six o'clock. Then six o'clock turned to six thirty, and it was getting dark fast. Every time I called Stephanie to check in with her, she was hysterical, crying on the street. To make matters worse, her children were growing hungry.

"Don't worry," I kept telling her in a reassuring tone that was a million miles away from what I was actually feeling. "We will find your mother."

I felt sure that Giuliana was indeed safe somewhere, but as the evening wore on, the temperature kept dropping, and it was too cold to be outside without a coat. I was concerned about the length of time it was taking to find her.

By seven o'clock, we had each covered about five miles as we walked slowly, peering around corners. Ginny, to whom I had given a visual description of Giuliana, walked patiently beside me the entire time, along with the dogs, who were of no help whatsoever, focused on enjoying the treat of an unexpectedly long walk. As time went on, I wondered how much longer Stephanie could wait before needing to take the ferry back to Staten Island. Right as I had started to feel quite hopeless, Ginny grabbed me with one hand and pointed with the other.

"Look!" she yelped excitedly. "Is that your

patient?"

Like a prayer answered, I saw the vision of an older woman peering determinedly into a mailbox a few feet away from us. We were exactly four blocks from my office.

I walked quickly over to Giuliana. "Hello," I said, trying to hide my relief and excitement.

"Hello," replied Giuliana with a bright smile, not recognizing me at all from earlier in the day. She was just naturally friendly. "It's cold out here."

"How are you doing?" I asked.

"Fine. How are you?" Giuliana responded, before turning to Ginny with a big smile. "Hello, bambina. How are you?"

I asked Giuliana where she had been.

"I had a coffee in a nice bakery," she said.

No wonder we hadn't been able to find her: While we were scouring the streets, she had been sitting in a café.

I thought to myself, *Not all who wander are lost.*

I called Stephanie, trying to mask the absolute relief I felt. After all, I had been telling her the entire time that her mother would be found.

"Your mother is right here on Park Avenue," I told Stephanie. "Meet us back at the office, and then you can all go home."

There was much rejoicing for Stephanie, but Giuliana had no sense that there had been any problem at all. She had no knowledge that she'd been lost. Once we got Giuliana wrapped up in her coat, she and Stephanie started the trip home to Staten Island. I headed home with my daughter and the dogs, thinking about what a tremendously stressful experience we had all had. It had been nerve-racking even for me, although I had no doubt that Giuliana would be found.

Losing Giuliana while she was in my care made me understand in a new, visceral way the urgency in caregivers' voices when they call me distressed about losing their loved one. It gave me a whole new understanding of what caregivers go through at home. When a person with dementia wanders off, it's deeply upsetting, but I try to tell caregivers that patients will just about always be found. They will manage to find their way home or seek appropriate help. Still, I understand how difficult this is to believe while the patient is missing.

On another occasion a patient who lived a few blocks from her daughter in Queens was supposed to drive to her daughter's for dinner, but never showed up. For hours through the night, my patient's daughter sat by the phone, frantically making calls to local hospitals and law enforcement, fearing the worst. She finally got a call from a gas station near Rochester, nearly three hundred miles away. It was her mother. It turned out she had become confused about the location of her daughter's house and had instead set off for her own childhood home in upstate New York. It was not until she ran low on fuel that she pulled into a gas station and asked for help.

Similarly, I remember when someone from a local television station called me one morning to arrange an afternoon interview with me because a celebrity with Alzheimer's — not my patient — was lost.

"She'll likely be found by then," I said. Happily, she was, and the interview was no longer necessary.

ANXIETY AS A CAUSE OF WANDERING BEHAVIOR

Another unusual incident in my office's history occurred with Jake, an athletic, wiry man of 78 with slowly progressive Alzheimer's disease, with mild-moderate memory loss and mild living skills and language loss. He had been divorced for fifteen years, but despite their long estrangement, his ex-wife had resurfaced after his diagnosis to take care of him. The ex–Mrs. Jake was a cool character, a tattooed biker chick with a busy life, but she couldn't bear the thought of her ex-husband trying to cope on his own. She let me know that he was becoming increasingly agitated and anxious, and we changed his medication to try to tackle these new problems.

Unfortunately, one afternoon, while we were still trying to figure out the right cocktail for him, Jake suddenly jumped up and ran out of my psychologist Casey's office. He was right in the middle of the brain exercise sessions that he usually enjoyed. In fact, Jake had grown very enamored of Casey, who had a caring and lovely manner with patients, so his abrupt exit was a big surprise.

Jake made it out of the office and past our doorman, and sped out into the city. Casey ran after him, but, alarmed, he responded physically, pushing her away.

"Leave me alone!" he yelled at the top of his lungs.

"It's all right, Jake," Casey replied. "I'm coming along with you for a walk."

Casey later told me that, despite her calm appearance, she was terrified that Jake would run out in the road and get hit by a car. I wished I had thought to tell her before then that patients with Alzheimer's are generally still careful and check for traffic before they cross the street, just as the rest of us do. It is an ingrained procedural memory skill for people who have lived in cities.

Jake, with Casey acting as his shadow, went along like this for a while, with Casey frantically sending frequent updates to the office from her cell phone. She told me that one of the worst things about the experience were the looks thrown her way by passersby, who didn't understand why Jake was screaming, "Stop abusing me! Stop beating me! Leave me alone!" Casey was a young psychologist at the time, and I believe the experience matured her considerably.

Jake and Casey got all the way up to 96th Street, an extremely busy thoroughfare, when Casey suddenly had the insight to try a covert method of redirection, which sometimes works with patients who are agitated and upset. Instead of continuing to follow Jake, she quickened her pace to walk directly in front of him. He automatically began to follow her, and when she took a left across 96th Street and came back down Lexington Avenue in the opposite direction, it was only natural for him to continue to trail her. This worked like a charm, even though Jake continued to yell at Casey the whole time. She quietly tried to reassure horrified strangers as they passed, mouthing, "It's okay, it's okay."

Jake followed Casey back to our office, not realizing that's what he was doing. On their return, Casey took him into her office and sat with him patiently until he calmed down.

Had Casey tried to confront Jake and prevent him from going forward on his path, he would have fought her, likely even pushed her out of his way. As it was, Casey understood that Jake was walking to reduce his sense of anxiety, so she instinctively did the best thing: She redirected him back toward our office while continuing to allow him to walk off his anxiety.

AN ER VISIT

Thankfully, I've had only one other wandering episode in my twenty-three years of practice. Bobby, a 68-year-old retired banker, walked out of my office during a split second when no one was watching him. By the time we discovered he was gone, we realized with horror that the last time anyone had seen him was nearly forty minutes earlier. Somehow, we had all assumed that his aide had picked him up and

335

taken him home. It wasn't until the aide finally arrived that we realized Bobby had left without our knowledge.

I called Bobby's wife, a woman of incredible strength who demonstrated a chronic inability to panic — a quality I admired now more than ever — to inform her that I had been remiss and that we had let Bobby leave the office.

"Bobby's lived in the city all his life and knows New York like the back of his hand," I told her. "He's probably walking back to your apartment."

"Yes," she agreed. "I'm not worried."

We waited, watching the clock tick along, with no sign of Bobby. When two hours had passed, Bobby's wife and I decided to start calling the local hospitals. She also called friends and relatives and a variety of other places she suspected he might show up.

Remarkably, we found Bobby in the hospital across the street from my office. Bobby had not only managed to get himself admitted, but had successfully acquired a bed for himself in the emergency department. He had done this in less than a half hour after leaving my office — quite a record, given how long emergency room visits usually take.

Bobby's wife and I rushed over to the

hospital to find him reclined comfortably in a bed, cool as a cucumber, with IVs running. He had already had blood drawn, and, for reasons that I couldn't fathom, X-rays taken. I asked the emergency room physician what had happened.

"Well," he said, shaking his head in puzzlement, "Bobby walked in and asked firmly, 'Who's in charge here?' Once he'd been directed to the head nurse, he gravely informed her that he was very sick and needed help. He was convincing enough to be admitted immediately — don't ask me how." We both laughed at the sheer unlikelihood of this, as we knew of numerous instances where far sicker patients were left languishing in emergency rooms waiting for assistance.

Knowing how effective and practical Bobby had been all of his life, this implausible scenario made perfect sense. Because he knew his name and date of birth, the hospital staff had been able to pull his old records. And because he had such presence, none of the ER personnel even suspected that he was on the Alzheimer's spectrum. They also had no idea that he was lost, and therefore made no attempt to contact his wife. The emergency room personnel did not notice the symptoms of Bobby's dementia. His wife signed him out against medical advice, because the hospital personnel thought he shouldn't be released until his laboratory tests had come back. I think Bobby probably set a record that day for the shortest processing period in a busy New York City emergency room.

To be able to take a jaunt out into the world, to be able to saunter around the block, to meander along in a park — these are simple and simply enormous joys of the freedom conferred by adulthood. Fear of the possibility of being lost or hurt prevents loving caregivers from allowing Alzheimer's patients to have this most basic of liberties: to let their legs take them places. Although there are, of course, sad exceptions to the rule, for the most part patients with Alzheimer's find their way back home or are found, safe and sound. Electronic aids and simpler tools like bracelets are invaluable both in allowing a patient freedom and relieving the caregiver's anxieties.

CHAPTER 11
I CAN'T TAKE IT ANYMORE!
ADVICE TO CAREGIVERS: SELF-CARE, STRESS REDUCTION, AND WHEN TO SEEK ADDITIONAL HELP

Chronic illness in the elderly is rising as more people live longer with infirmities. Alzheimer's is the most rapidly growing category, but many other illnesses, such as cancer, heart disease, and strokes, also require significant amounts of caregiving. Family members make up the majority of caregivers, and spouses make up the majority of this group. Most people don't have any training in being caregivers and are thrown into the role. It's not an easy job for anyone, and it's particularly tough on spouses, because the job is round-the-clock, every day of the year.

Being the spouse caregiver for someone on the Alzheimer's spectrum can be the loneliest role of their life — the spouse is caring for the person they are closest to and whose support they need the most, even as that person is not as available to be supportive. Long-term relationships are often grounded in one person taking care of certain activities and the other attending to others — for example, one spouse enjoying cooking, the other driving; one taking care of bookkeeping, the other the garden. These roles become upended, with the caregiver assuming many if not all the duties of the couple. Caregivers have to manage not only their own lives, but also the lives of the loved one with Alzheimer's. This is not a task for which they receive much thanks. The patient may resist being told what to do, family members may criticize the caregiver, friends may stay away. . . . It is a lonely, lonely place to be. It is no wonder that more than half of all caregivers of patients with dementia suffer from depression and anxiety. I try my best to help caregivers survive this time — triumph over it, even — and that begins with one thing: putting the caregiver's needs first.

This is not selfishness or self-serving behavior. This is about Survival Over the Long Haul, about doing what is best for both the patient and the caregiver. All that tremendous loneliness, exhaustion, and sadness can be at least partially alleviated with small changes in attitude and behavior. The first and most important thing that I counsel caregivers to let go of is guilt: guilt for not spending enough time with the patient, guilt for not being patient enough or stimulating enough, guilt for yearning to escape — the list is endless. As in the rest of life, one's approach toward caregiving can help shape the experience — how we frame an experience colors our enjoyment of it.

THE IDEAL CAREGIVER

Martin was an anomaly, the rare caregiver who had it all going on, accepting his role with grace and humor — even enjoying it. I believe this was because his innate personality traits lent themselves perfectly to the role he found himself in. He was an inherently practical man, loyal, and not prone to guilt, and he delegated well. He had few expectations of his children and could laugh about the lighter side of things even when life got heavy. He had picked up additional coping skills from a lifetime spent as an athletic coach. He was one of my favorite caregivers ever, someone whom I admired and adored — thinking about him brings a smile to my face to this day.

Martin's approach to caregiving was sensitive, but also matter-of-fact. He cheerfully was able to accept a huge responsibility without developing feelings of resentment. He started out taking care of his wife, Lisa, by himself, but recognized when things began getting too tough to handle on his own and hired a caregiver to help him out. He kept in close contact with their four grown children but did not require actual hands-on caregiving from them, saying, "They all have their lives, their jobs, their kids." He spent time with his friends a few days a week. Best of all, he maintained his sense of humor.

Lisa, who had slowly progressive Alzheimer's disease, became my patient when I was still a newbie in the field. Martin chose me as her neurologist after "shopping around" because he found that I was more interested in supporting caregivers than the other doctors he had seen. As the years went by, he was fond of repeating, "I knew when we first met you, you were the one for Lisa and me. We are a team, and you saw us as a team. You didn't dismiss Lisa, and you saw what was important to me. I felt like you were looking out not just for her, but for the two of us."

Martin had an easy, fun-loving way with everyone and particularly with Lisa. He joked around with her and teased her without being demeaning. Because of his coaching background, Martin was prone to saying such things as "C'mon, Speedy! Let's get going!" to his wife as she tottered around. This usually made her giggle.

I loved Martin's manner with his wife. He was completely devoted to her but didn't take himself or the situation too seriously. He could coax her to do things without being too "managerial," and he never lost sight of the fact that he was her husband first and her caregiver second. "I so admire you, Martin," I'd tell him. "You're an inspiration to us all."

"What do you want me to do?" he would exclaim. "Sit down and cry over it? No way, José! Lisa spent all her life taking care of me and our kids. She helped out with the business when things were slow. This is the least I can do." Then he'd turn to her and say, "Isn't that right, Speedy?" and she would look at him and smile.

When Martin left for the supermarket, Lisa would wait at the window for him, like a forlorn pet.

"My heart sinks when I see her looking at me through the window," he would tell me. "I know she doesn't want me to leave, but I have to run these errands. I tell her on the way out, 'Speedy, I'll be right back!' and I make an effort to be as fast as possible."

I asked him how he managed being with her with no escape — how he managed not to feel trapped. He always laughed his larger-than-life laugh and said, "Lisa and I have had a wonderful life. We still have a pretty good life. We have moments, but who doesn't?"

Several years later, a few weeks after Lisa died, Martin stopped by my office for an unannounced visit, bringing with him a large crocheted patchwork blanket. "Lisa was always talking about making you something, but she never got around to it, so I am giving you this. She made this when our daughter was bedridden. She sat up every night for six months, taking care of Lily, and I didn't hear her complain once. You remember you asked me once why I didn't feel trapped? How was I going to complain because she didn't want me to leave her? It's about for better or worse, in sickness and in health, right? We were together in this, Speedy and me, and now she's gone."

I still have the blanket, my present from Lisa and Martin. I love it because the wool and the vibrant colors warm me on cold winter nights, but even more because crocheted into it is Lisa and Martin's story. Martin was a great caregiver not only because he knew how to take care of his wife — which many caregivers do — but also because he knew how to *take care of himself,* which few caregivers seem to know how to do.

ANGELA — A MORE
TYPICAL CAREGIVER

In contrast to Martin, Angela was having a far more difficult time. She was the wife of my patient Ed, who at 78 had had Alzheimer's for six years. One day, she walked into my office and exploded.

"I can't stand it anymore!" she exclaimed. "If Ed tells me he loves me one more time, I'm going to have to kill him."

I looked at her and didn't say a word, listening.

"He follows me everywhere," she explained. "I don't have a moment to myself. When I go to the bathroom and shut the door, he knocks to make sure I'm there. When I open the door, he's standing there, waiting for me. Sometimes, when I run out to do a quick errand, he's going crazy by the time I come home. Even when I leave reminders of where I am, he forgets to look for them and paces up and down our front porch, waiting for me. He's even wandered over to our neighbors' houses, looking for me.

"Sometimes," Angela continued, "I want to scream, 'Don't you know I'm here? I only left for five minutes!' But he looks at me and says, 'I love you so much. You're so good to me,' and I don't know what to do."

Frantic anxiety in patients when their caregiver is out of sight is a common problem. Although it's more typical when the spouse or child is the caregiver, it can also occur with paid help to whom the patient has become attached. Such anxiety frequently creates internal conflict within the caregiver, because even though they understand that the strength of the bond between them has caused their loved one to become almost physically attached to them, they also yearn to break free and find some space to breathe. They experience guilt for desiring any alone time, even if it's just to sit quietly and read. The caregiver is in an emotional and physical pressure cooker with little way to let off steam. This can ultimately create a situation where the caregiver becomes aggressive toward the patient, either verbally or physically or both.

As Angela explained the situation, I could imagine her and Ed enacting the typical scenes that play out in caregiver-patient duos.

"Stop it!" Angela screams. "Ed, why don't

you stop it, for heaven's sake! I am in the bathroom!"

"I am sorry," Ed responds, his face close to the other side of the bathroom door. "I'm sorry, honey. I love you."

Angela, overcome by guilt, love, and the trap she finds herself in, breaks into quiet tears of frustration, anger, and sadness. On the other side of the door, I imagine Ed getting worried, because there is no sound from his wife on the inside.

"Angela," I asked her now, "do you get to spend any time by yourself, doing things you enjoy? Do you ever go get a manicure, get your hair done, or spend time with your friends?"

"I'd like to have some me time," Angela answered. "But Ed doesn't like to lose sight of me. I am not much of a manicure gal, but I used to sing with my church choir three evenings a week. I enjoyed that, but I had to give it up. I used to have brunch with my girlfriends on Saturdays at the mall, but that also had to go. Ed drives me crazy, but I can't leave him home by himself. He misses me so."

I have heard about many emotionally draining scenes like this one — they can play out several times a day, every day, in the lives of couples like Angela and Ed.

I eventually persuaded Angela to hire some outside help to stay with her husband a few evenings a week so she could return to choir practice. She was initially reluctant, because she felt guilty enjoying herself when Ed was home waiting for her. I also prescribed medication for Ed's anxiety to help make their separations less painful for them both. They reached an uneasy status quo, primarily because Angela continued to feel guilty about not being a "good" wife by leaving Ed alone and spending time caring for herself.

Not all of my patients on the Alzheimer's spectrum develop Ed's kind of separation anxiety. Many continue to live contented lives, without disquiet. For patients who do develop such anxieties, fortunately effective treatment exists in the form of medication, as we discussed in Chapter 8; I'm in favor of treatment being sought *before* the caregiver reaches their breaking point.

I see many caregivers like Angela — depressed and completely burned out but unwilling to get help, consumed by guilt and anger at the same time. Having more time to herself would have not only helped Angela feel less depressed but made her less angry and irritable with Ed. Alas, Angela's sense of duty and code of ethics did not allow for such an approach.

ANOTHER KIND OF
SEPARATION ANXIETY

My patient Sarah and her husband, Paul, had not spent a day apart in their sixty-plus years of marriage, hard as that may be to believe. Now retired, Paul had been a very successful physician and Sarah had managed his office. Even after she developed Alzheimer's, he doted on her and showered her with gifts. He would buy her gorgeous stockings because, even in her eighties, she loved wearing fine hosiery that showed off her toned calves. Sarah's internist, who had been Paul's medical student, said admiringly, "They are like Tracy and Hepburn."

One morning Paul came into my office with a tragic look on his face. I asked him what had happened.

"I can't believe what I did," he said, forlorn.

I asked again what had happened.

"I've never raised a hand against Sarah before," Paul said. "She followed me into the library one too many times and — I don't know what came over me — I reached out and I tried to choke her." He lifted up his hands, staring at them with disbelief.

Then he dropped them helplessly down to his sides.

Utterly distraught, he broke down in tears. "I love Sarah! She is my life! But I don't have any space, any time to myself. She follows me everywhere like a puppy," he said, sobbing. "Yesterday, she soiled the couch again, even though I'd taken her to the bathroom several times to make sure she didn't have an accident. She doesn't like to wear diapers, so I don't put her in Depends, so I had to clean that couch for the second time this month."

Paul was in his late eighties and slightly built, and it was hard to watch his small frame shake with sobs. I realized that I was serving in the role of priest — I was listening to a confession.

"You're not the first person who's done this, and you won't be the last," I told Paul, trying to offer him some comfort, some absolution. I knew that he was a gentle man and that he would never seriously hurt his wife; he was simply at his breaking point and needed help.

"Taking care of your wife, by yourself, at home — that's an enormous responsibility," I continued. "You bathe her, feed her, spend the whole day with her, and take her out to movies and the museum to keep her alert.

Then you come home and you sleep next to her. If you didn't get angry with her every once in a while, you wouldn't really be human."

I tried to convey to him that he wasn't a monster for doing what he did, that I was positive he wouldn't do it again, and that it was very brave for him to come in and talk to me honestly about it. I knew he was actually asking for help with his situation, a situation that was precipitated by his wife being so needy of his physical presence. I prescribed a low dose of an antidepressant, antianxiety medication for Sarah, which reduced her fearfulness when she was apart from her husband. I also referred Sarah to a local senior day program to give Paul a bit of a break, but in an ironic twist, it didn't work the way I expected — because Paul enrolled as well and sat with her! It turned out Paul had a bit of separation anxiety himself.

Although it would be nice to think that Paul might have had some relief at the center, where staff members were around, he couldn't get rid of his inner physician self. He thought he knew what was best for Sarah, hovered over her constantly, and did not allow the staff to help in any substantive way. After a month of this, we gave up on the senior center for the Paul and Sarah team.

Eventually Paul agreed to bring in a paid aide to help alleviate some of his stress by taking on some of his caregiving responsibilities. Sarah's anxiety was further diminished by the presence of the aide, someone with whom she came to feel very comfortable. This allowed Paul to spend a few hours on his own each day, reading his medical journals and going to the hospital to say hello to his old colleagues. He regained a sense of himself as someone other than a caregiver. These short periods apart ultimately enabled Paul to be a superior and less angry caregiver.

Although separation anxiety can create the type of clinging behavior in patients that increases caregiver stress, there are obviously many other causes of stress as well. Financial uncertainty, the inability to work, social isolation, lack of support, feeling misunderstood or unappreciated by not only the patient but by other family members as well — the list goes on and on.

When the stress gets to be too much and the caregiver explodes, it understandably creates tremendous feelings of guilt. All too often, the caregiver suffers alone with it. They quietly loathe themselves, despite the fact that they are trapped in an often thankless, lonely, 24/7 job from which it seems like there is no escape. Even on vacation with the patient, they're still taking care of a person who, day by day, may be becoming progressively more dependent.

For those who want to be helpful to caregivers, I have three words of advice: Support, Support, Support. Not criticism, not remonstration, not "how could you do that?!" but Support, with a capital *S*. That is what caregivers need most, as we saw with both Paul and Angela, and it's the mantra I recite in all my caregiver interactions. The Alzheimer's Association has an extensive national network of free support groups for caregivers where they can share stories, feel less alone, and learn techniques to help better care for themselves and for loved ones on the spectrum.

FINDING JOY IN THE CAREGIVING THICKET

Oftentimes, the caregiving aspects of the relationship tend to overwhelm the spousal aspects of it. Martin knew how to balance the two roles, but Angela did not. It's important to carve out one-on-one time to enjoy the patient as a person, without the specter of illness hanging over every moment. Being able to do this allowed Martin to continue to enjoy Lisa's company and helped Paul enjoy Sarah's company once again.

This communion can be achieved in many ways. Some patients are fond of hiking or bridge or golf or gardening, activities that the caregiver could enjoy with them. Some love listening to music, and others take pleasure in cooking. Meaningful interaction can occur even with patients at the severe end of the spectrum.

My 90-year-old patient Camille was fifteen years into her mildly progressive Alzheimer's. She needed help with eating, dressing, toileting, and walking, so her husband of almost seven decades, Andrew, had hired help during the day. Nonetheless, Andrew felt helpless and despondent as Camille got worse. She desperately needed more exercise to keep from becoming chair bound.

I discovered that both Andrew and Camille enjoyed dancing, so I suggested that they dance together for a half hour each day. Not only did this help Camille keep up her strength, but the activity brought them both joy. Andrew particularly enjoyed their "danceathons" as he called them — they were a source of great sustenance to him.

"We waltzed to 'Moon River' last week,"

he said recently, and laughed. "It was such fun — brought back old memories. Camille has always been a good dancer." Dancing allowed him to reconnect with his wife and made him feel like he was helping her at the same time.

SCHEDULING BREAKS

The trick for each caregiver is to find out what makes them tick — what offers them pleasure and relaxes them, what restores them — and *schedule* time for it. I'm a big believer in caregivers taking not just the occasional vacation but breaks *every day,* so they have restorative time for themselves on a regular basis. In other words, they shouldn't put breaks off until the end of the month, the end of the year, or some nebulous time in the future, but should schedule in a mini-break every day, whether that means taking a walk, getting a pedicure, or rolling around on the carpet with the dog.

Actually scheduling in the "me time" is important, because otherwise, in my experience, it invariably gets postponed or doesn't happen, as there is always another caregiving chore beckoning around the corner. Of course, longer vacations are wonderful, but only if they allow a break from caregiving — in other words, if someone else is available to help alleviate the caregiving burden. Without personal time, burnout will happen, whether you are a family member or paid caregiver.

One evening, walking through Central Park, I ran into the wife of a former patient. Gwen was in her early sixties, tall and hearty, with closely cropped white hair framing a cheery face. She and her husband, Tom, had moved to Arizona a few years earlier.

"What are you doing back in New York?" I asked, pleased to see her.

"Remember what you told me about having weekends away from Tom every month? This is my weekend off, and here I am in New York, having a grand old time!" she said.

We both burst out laughing, because we realized how far we'd come from the early days, when I had to plead with Gwen to take even an afternoon off from caring for her husband. Tom suffered from advanced Parkinson's disease, and it meant that he was almost completely dependent on Gwen.

"That would be deserting him," she used to say. "I can't do that to him."

"But Gwen," I would implore, "it's important for you. You're taking care of him all day, every day. You need some time off."

Eventually, I persuaded her to take one evening a week for herself while her son came in and looked after Tom. By the time they moved to Arizona, I had persuaded Gwen to take a scheduled monthly break of two to four days. She found a paid caregiver whom she trusted to spend that time with Tom, and she would meet her girlfriends and go to a spa, or visit with her family in California. Surprisingly for Gwen, she eventually took to these forced vacations with enthusiasm. I was pleased to see her in New York, blooming and smiling.

"I come out here every few months," Gwen explained. "I miss my friends back East, and it's nice to get away from home."

"How is Tom?" I asked.

"He's doing as well as he can," Gwen said. "We're taking care of him at home. He and I wouldn't have it any other way, as you know."

As we parted ways, I had a small smile of satisfaction on my face. I was pleased to see Gwen in such good spirits, because I believed that the happier Gwen was, and the more respite she had, the more patient a caregiver and wife she would be with Tom, and the happier he would be.

Every time the caregiver of a patient takes time off, I consider it a small victory, not only for myself and for the caregiver, but also for my patient. This is because I know that the caregiver will have a little more tolerance for my patient's repetitions and be less prone to snap, and there will be a little more richness in the relationship between the two of them.

THE GLASS HALF FULL

It's understandable for caregivers who are friends and family to mourn aspects of the person that they've lost, but there's still a lot of the individual there — you just have to search a little harder than you did before to find him or her. This is particularly important in Alzheimer's disease, where the caregiver may be losing the treasured emotional support of the person they are caring for just when they need it most. A husband who relied on his wife to help cheer him up during difficult times, and whose advice he valued, no longer has access to that counsel and cheer when he needs it most. It can be quite lonely, but there are ways of making it better.

Laura, my patient Levi's wife, found a way. Both had been high-powered attorneys, and Laura was still working in her practice. Levi was now 84 with Lewy body dementia, another common type of dementia, and had been under my care for more than eleven years. During this time, he had had all available treatments, and although his dementia progressed, I believe it was far more gradual than it would have been without treatment. He still worked out at the gym, but he had become much quieter. When Laura got home from work, she now spent more time with caregiving activities, helping Levi with bathing and self-care.

Yet whenever I saw them together, Laura always treated Levi like her husband and partner, rather than her charge. She was consistently respectful and kind. I asked Laura how she maintained her respect for her husband in the face of the dementia.

"When Levi first showed symptoms, I was a crazy lady; I couldn't handle his behavior," she said, referring to Levi's impulsivity, poor judgment, agitation, and anxiety at the time of his diagnosis. Fortunately, these symptoms responded to medication and abated.

"I threatened to leave him," she continued. "I couldn't wrap my head around his crazy behavior. But at some point, I calmed down. I realized Levi is still Levi. He has remained such a sweet man. Even all these years later, he has a good quality of life. He still goes to the gym every day, he enjoys his meals and music, and we watch TV together.

"Maybe it's the way I approach life — I'm not that analytical," she added. "I could look at the husband I lost, but I choose to look at the man I still have and love."

I think Laura has been able to maintain this view because she has additional caregiving help that has allowed her to continue to work. This prevents her role from being winnowed down to that of "caregiver" alone, which is the fate of many caregivers, particularly women. Her full life allows her to savor her intimacy with Levi in the evenings. They have dinner together. They watch their favorite shows. They hold hands. These seemingly small interactions allow for self-replenishment, both for Levi and for Laura. Laura's weekday responsibilities give her time to nurture herself, to be someone other than a caregiver, and that provides her the emotional resources to continue to see her husband as the man she loved and married. In general, I have found that caregivers who work or routinely spend time apart from the patient for another reason report more life satisfaction and more joy in their interactions with the patient.

Advice to Caregivers
Here are a few recommendations for caregivers of Alzheimer's patients that will help

prevent burnout.

- Take a break, *every single day,* even if it's just a stroll around the block. Leaving a patient with Alzheimer's alone so you can have time to yourself doesn't make you negligent.

- Don't lose your loved one for the disease. You are the spouse, child, or partner, *not* the physical therapist, nurse, or taskmaster. Find ways to maintain a sense of closeness and connectedness.

- Introduce in-home care — present it as help for yourself if the patient refuses. In nearly all states, Medicare and Medicaid pay for a few hours of weekly care for patients with dementia.

- Remember there are two levels of communication — respond to the subtext. Logic may not be useful.

- You are not a saint — you will get angry and have a range of negative emotions. That's okay.

- Take care of your needs — have a cup of tea and read the paper, get a massage or a haircut, pursue your hobbies, spend time with friends. This is not being selfish; it is being smart about caregiving. Remember, when the pressure drops in an airplane cabin, the instructions are always to place the oxygen mask on yourself first before helping others.

• Join an Alzheimer's or dementia caregiver support group. They are free and run by groups such as the Alzheimer's Association.

WHEN TO GET PAID HELP

Juan, 73, was a devoted caregiver to his wife, Carolina, 72, who had raised their kids while he worked as a plumber. I had diagnosed Carolina with rapidly progressive Alzheimer's disease with mild memory impairment and moderate language impairment when she was 62. In addition to oral medications, Carolina did a few sessions of transcranial magnetic stimulation (TMS). We enrolled her in a clinical trial, and Juan drove his wife from their home in Queens to a university hospital in Pennsylvania every few weeks for two years. Although the treatments helped to slow the progression of her Alzheimer's, Carolina still got gradually worse. Ten years after her diagnosis, Juan found himself keeping house, cooking, bathing her, doing her nails, and toileting her.

Juan had a temper, and sometimes he would lash out at Carolina in frustration. Every now and again, when she came in to see me, I would see black and blue bruises

362

on her from when Juan had tried to move her or lift her too roughly.

"She won't stand still!" he would yell when I asked about it.

"Juan, I know you love Carolina," I would tell him, "but you need help."

"We're not ready for that yet, Doc," Juan would respond. "I'll let you know when we're ready."

"But Juan!" I protested, noting his ever-expanding frame, "you're putting on weight, you're stressed out, and you're in your sixties. What if you had a heart attack? What would happen to Carolina then?"

"I would take her with me to the hospital, Doc."

Juan refused to take my advice. As time passed, the woes kept piling on, and I reached the point where I'd dread their visits because I didn't know what might have happened since the previous one — it was rarely good. I was worried that at some point, Juan would do something to hurt Carolina, even though he loved her very much.

Early one Friday morning, I got a call from my answering service. Juan had paged them, something he had never done before in our ten-year relationship. He was on the phone, sobbing.

"I can't do it anymore, Doc," he cried. "I can't. I've reached the end. I cannot do it anymore."

That morning, Juan had tried to get Carolina off the toilet and they had both fallen to the bathroom floor. With neither of them physically fit enough to get up, this left Juan and Carolina stranded on the wet and dirty floor until he was eventually able to gather enough strength to crawl to the telephone and get help from a neighbor.

"I don't want to put her in a home," Juan said, sighing. "I have never wanted to. But I simply can't deal with it anymore."

"Juan, this is exactly what I was afraid of," I told him. "You don't want to put her in a home, she doesn't want to be in a home, but you've set up the situation so there's no other option. I wish you'd give me a few weeks to come up with an alternative. At that time, if it doesn't work, I promise I will help you in whatever way I can to find Carolina a good nursing home."

Eventually, Juan reluctantly agreed. Through their church, we found Erica, a brisk, no-nonsense woman originally from Jamaica who, at 75, was older than both Juan and Carolina. However, she was in great shape. She moved into the basement apartment in their house and cared for

Carolina while Juan continued to work.

"I'm a vegetarian," Erica informed me, when she came in for a visit with Carolina and Juan. A vibrant woman, she was responding to my question about how she kept herself so trim. "Are you a vegetarian? That's the way to good health. That, and the good Lord."

Initially, I worried about her compatibility with Carolina and Juan, who were both immigrants from Spain and had spent all their adult lives in Queens, but it was a match made in heaven. Erica turned out to be exactly what Juan needed. She took care of shopping, housekeeping, and bathing Carolina. When Juan came home from work, there was Carolina, bathed and "sweet smelling." Juan told me he was more in love with Carolina than he had ever been.

Fast-forward two years, and they are all still in the house together — Erica in the basement, Juan and Carolina upstairs. Both Carolina and Juan have lost weight eating the healthful vegetarian meals that Erica prepares. Carolina has remained relatively stable, still enjoying life. Juan told me that between Carolina's Social Security and her pension, and his job, they have remained financially comfortable. He realized that, in addition to everyone being happier, it was less expensive to keep Carolina at home than to place her in a nursing home.

Recently, I received an email from Juan. "I love Carolina and I love Erica," Juan declared. "Erica is the most beautiful woman in my life! Thank you." Who would've thunk it? I was pleased as punch.

How to Find Paid Caregiver Help

Before you start looking for someone, think about exactly what you would like the caregiver to do, how many hours and days a week you need them, and whether they would live in or live out. A thorough interview is essential. In addition to conscientiousness, kindness, and reliability, a crucial caregiver characteristic is compatibility with the patient. Although finding the right person may seem like a daunting task, there are organizations that can help. Here are a few places to consider:

- Professional caregiving agencies
- Churches and religious organizations
- Local universities with students looking for part-time employment
- Professional societies such as the Screen Actors Guild or special-interest support groups such as SAGE — Seniors Aging in a Gay Environment
- Local senior centers or dementia physi-

cians, who sometimes have lists of interested people
• Local Alzheimer's Association chapters, which may maintain lists of agencies

And don't forget to ask around in your apartment building and neighborhood — you may be able to find someone who lives nearby who would be happy to have a job helping out. Many of my patients have found good and reliable help in this fashion.

WHEN PATIENTS REFUSE PAID CAREGIVING HELP

In Juan and Carolina's case, it was Juan who resisted having a paid caregiver, but more often, it's the patients themselves who resist. Many absolutely refuse to have a caregiver or simply fire everybody who's hired. Even when the patient has more advanced dementia, he or she might still refuse a caregiver's help, despite the family's pleas. Eventually, the family throws up their hands in frustration and lets the caregiver go.

Caregivers may also quit because of the unpleasantness of the interactions with the patient. Although it is understandably wearying to be the target of hostility and even accusations, experienced caregivers know enough not to take it personally.

Oftentimes they can even allow themselves to be "fired" and return quietly an hour later to a patient who has forgotten the fight.

It often takes a little imagination to find the right way to explain the presence of a caregiver to a patient. I remember one situation where things spiraled out of control. Bettina was a widow who lived alone in Brooklyn. Now retired, she had been in charge of a secretarial pool and was accustomed to bossing people around. Her two daughters lived out of state and took turns bringing their mother to my office, flying in specifically for the appointments.

"I don't understand why you put me on these pills," Bettina would say to me, convinced that her memory was still perfect. "There's nothing wrong with me. There's something wrong with her!" And with that, she would point her thumb accusingly at whichever daughter was accompanying her. When this happened, Bettina's daughters would sigh and shake their heads.

Because of her forgetfulness, Bettina failed to take not just her Alzheimer's medicine but her other medications as well, and as a result, her blood pressure and her diabetes were poorly controlled. She was constantly confused, not just because of her dementia, but also because of her wildly fluctuating blood sugar and blood pressure levels. Because of the poor blood pressure control, she was very much at risk for a stroke, which would further worsen her dementia.

At home, Bettina often didn't have enough food because she forgot to stock up regularly. When it snowed, she insisted on shoveling her driveway by herself, sometimes while wearing her nightgown. Bettina's neighbors became concerned. Finally, despite her protests that she was fine on her own, her daughters hired caregivers to look after their mom, but Bettina fired each of them, frequently with a wrongful accusation that they were stealing from her.

It got to the point where I began sending my nurse to see Bettina every week, to help ensure that she was taking her medications. We figured out a whole system of Monday–Sunday pillboxes, but Bettina simply threw them away and tried to find the pills in their original bottles. Because we had removed them, she would go to the pharmacist and make a fuss until she got new medications.

Eventually, we found a caregiver who was compatible with Bettina. Megan was the same age, the widowed sister of a neighbor. She had found herself in financial straits as the result of pension fund mismanagement and a foreclosure on her home. When

Megan moved in, she did so under the guise of someone who needed both work and a place to stay. She presented herself as someone who needed help. This appeased Bettina's pride and allowed her to feel like someone who was doing the caring, rather than the person being cared for. Bettina found the situation appealing, because she had always enjoyed taking care of people.

Bettina didn't know that this new guest in her home was being surreptitiously paid by her daughters. She assumed that Megan was providing housekeeping help because she was getting a place to stay rent-free. Bettina would bring Megan along to her visits to my office and explain to me, "Well, Megan needed help, and you know I like to try to help everyone."

Bettina's symptoms stabilized with Megan's oversight of her medications and with her companionship. She has continued to live at home and enjoy a good quality of life.

CAREGIVER COMPATABILITY

One reason for Bettina and Megan's compatible pairing was that they were of similar background, but as we saw with Erica and Carolina, this is not always a requirement. However, when a patient is embarrassed about the need for caregiving, a caregiver of a different race or one who is significantly younger is harder to "pass off" as a friend or family member. In such cases, if the caregiver is of the same social, cultural, and/or racial background, the patient may feel more comfortable in public settings. These are realities we have to contend with, and I try to discuss that as openly as possible.

I recently was chatting with a patient with migraines whose mother had Alzheimer's but was flatly refusing help. My patient asked for advice about ways to persuade her mother to accept the care she needed.

"You know, it's not uncommon for patients to refuse help," I told her, before giving her a list of agencies whose caregivers had experience with patients with Alzheimer's.

"Well, there's an additional problem, Dr. Devi," my patient confessed in embarrassment. "My mom has become very racist."

"That's not uncommon either," I told her. "Some patients may want to be with someone who's like them, and race can be a component of that." This is an uncomfortable and painful issue to raise in our society. Although bigotry in any form is not to be condoned, the patient's comfort level needs to be factored in. Additional sources of bias can include age, sex, class, and education. The paid caregiver should be someone with whom the patient feels compatible and connected.

All that said, it's hard to predict what will work best, and sometimes you have to rely on trial and error. One of my patients, Don, a retired army general in his nineties, went through a series of caregivers whom he kept firing, much to his wife's frustration. A service agency tried every combination of live-in caregiver, including a retired veteran in his fifties. No go. After a few days, Don would show them the door. The person Don, who was white, finally settled on was Evan, a 28-year-old, gay, African American actor with tattoos. Although Evan had no formal caregiving training, he had a natural empathy and intelligence, and he and Don clicked. He had an easy, relaxed way about him and never tired of hearing Don's World War II stories. He lived in one of the spare bedrooms in Don and his wife's apartment for two years until Don died. He had a rent-free space and time off for auditions and performances, as well as a steady salary. Toward the end of their time together, the unlikely duo of Evan and Don even went to Florida and played some golf, leaving Don's wife back at home to enjoy a few days to herself.

Don and Evan's story illustrates that ultimately the arrangements that work best are those in which the personalities of the caregiver and patient are complementary. Bettina was bossy and Megan was willing to be bossed around, which made their relationship work. Don loved to tell stories and Evan was a good listener. Juan and Carolina were steak-and-beer folks and Erica was a vegetarian, but they shared common religious and family values. Although similar backgrounds are sometimes important, much more often it is the personality fit and the level of respect in the relationship between the patient and the caregiver that is crucial.

THE VALUE OF STAYING AT HOME

When caregiving duties become overwhelming and paid caregivers are not an option, placing the patient in a facility seems to be an obvious solution. Unfortunately, such placement does not always solve the problems it seems like it would solve. Recent research suggests that families of patients who have put their loved ones in nursing homes experience new and different forms of stress. This is brought about by many factors relating to the move, including, but not limited to, guilt about "abandoning" loved ones, difficulty interacting with professional caregivers at the new facility (who may have differing ideas about how best to take care of individual patients), and the burden of having to travel (sometimes relatively long, time-consuming distances) to see the patient.

Finally, and perhaps most important, research has shown that many long-term caregivers who ultimately put their loved one into a professional facility still find it difficult to let go of the commitment they feel to the patient's care. This can result in them continuing to spend their days with the patient and performing the same tasks they did at home, including bathing, feeding, and toileting — only now, they are performing those tasks in an environment that is alien for the patient and inconvenient for the caregiver.

While we are focusing on the caregiver perspective in this chapter, I should say that one of the major fears voiced by many of my patients after they have received a diagnosis on the Alzheimer's spectrum is that they will be "shipped off" to a nursing home by their families. In fact, this is a deterrent to some patients seeking help, because they believe that an Alzheimer's label is synonymous with being sent to a home. More often than not, patients may nurse this fear in secret, and their anxiety may manifest in inexplicable behaviors that begin to make sense once this fear is understood. Patients may vehemently refuse help with activities where they clearly might need help, such as with taking pills regularly or getting dressed in seasonally appropriate clothing.

"I know what she wants to do," my patient Bernadette, who had Alzheimer's, confessed to me about her daughter Radha's offers to help. "She'll take over the bills, then the housework, and then it's off to the nursing home for me. I have to stop her from taking over."

When I mentioned this to Radha, she burst out laughing. "Oh my God, now it makes so much sense why Mom has been behaving like a nut! I had no idea."

Once Radha reassured her mother that she had no intention of putting her in a home, Bernadette was more accepting of help. In my experience, such reassurance needs to be ongoing. At the very outset, when the diagnosis is discussed with the patient and family, I make it a point to stress that the goal of treatment is to live functionally and at home. Some patients are terrified that if they even let the words *nursing home* escape their lips, their family members will move faster in that direction. Giving voice to the dreaded words is a good way to begin the conversation about this difficult and barely-spoken-of topic — the elephant in the room for many Alzheimer's patients — even in those cases where ultimately the result may be placement.

MY IDEAL NURSING HOME — AN INTERGENERATIONAL UTOPIA

Although I'm a huge proponent of keeping patients with dementia at home, for those times when a nursing home is unavoidable, my ideal facility would be a place where young folk and the elderly commingle. I believe that this type of interaction can't help but improve the quality of life for all concerned. Intergenerational exchanges bring purpose and meaning into the life of an elderly person and love and patience into the life of a child. Such places do exist. Sited at a senior care center, a preschool in Seattle is breaking through our society's increasing generational segregation. The preschoolers and seniors join together for activities such as music, art, and storytelling. A nursing home in Japan operates on a similar concept. There is much that the elderly and the young can gain from each other.

I remember the words of a dear friend and patient, who died at the age of 101 and was fond of wearing a white carnation in his buttonhole. He would tell me, "Gayatri, make sure you have friends from every decade of your life. That keeps you from getting lonely as you get older."

He developed a wonderful relationship with my daughter, whom he met when she was 11 and he was in his late eighties. For a birthday, he sent her a little whistle pendant, along with a card that said, "Whistle and I will come." My daughter wrote back a thank-you note that said, "If *you* whistle, *I* will come." Such lively banter between two people separated by nearly seventy years is heartwarming.

Growing up, I spent a lot of time with my grandparents, as my parents were busy with their professional lives. One grandmother taught me how to read, and the other taught me how to cook. One grandfather took me on long walks and taught me to enjoy nature. The other taught me how to be assertive and in charge. They had more time, affection, and wisdom to share than my parents did at that busy period of their young adult lives. I find this generosity of time and knowledge in my patients as well. What a shame it would be to sequester such richness within the confines of a facility.

The sad truth is that such intergenerational facilities are few and far between for a multitude of reasons, including legal liabilities and acceptance by society at large. When choosing a nursing home, one should ideally opt for a site that most resembles the place the loved one lives in and enjoys, rather than proximity to family. If a patient has lived their whole life in a rural community, for instance, moving them to a facility in a large city to be closer to a daughter and her children is not ideal for the patient (although it may be for his daughter). Moving into a place where friends and neighbors of the patient are also living would be good. My friend Amy's parents were lucky in the place they were able to find.

FINDING UTOPIA IN WISCONSIN

Amy, born and raised in rural Wisconsin, moved to New York City for college and stayed, choosing to marry and raise her own children in the metropolis. Her parents, with whom she was close, hated the city when they visited, much as they doted on their only child. As they grew older, Amy fretted about how they would manage during the harsh winters they experienced in their large home in a small farming town.

In their midseventies, her parents and a whole bunch of friends from their church signed up together for an assisted-living-to-nursing-home facility that was being built close by. As a group, they sold their houses and moved into the facility. The place had daily activities, bus trips to different venues, and a large on-site guesthouse for visiting family. Amy visited with her children and told me in surprise, "I have never liked the idea of those places, but my parents seem happy here. It's like a Lutheran resort! They have their friends with them, they don't have to worry about going to the super-market if they don't feel like it, and I don't have to worry that Dad is going to break his leg trying to repair the roof.

"It's kind of like a senior dorm," she said. "When they lived at home, they got on each other's nerves sometimes, particularly in the winter when it was hard to visit with their friends. Here they have their own cliques.

"My mom is part of the same clique she was in back in high school, although I don't know if that is good or bad," she added, laughing.

Amy's parents were lucky that they had a community of friends who together had the foresight to plan for the future. I hope more and more people do the same.

Her parents grew old with the friends they had known all their lives. When someone in their group needed more care because of cognitive or medical difficulties, they were placed in higher-level facilities in the same compound, a kind of aging in place. Another kind of Eden, it is all in the eyes of the beholder.

A Serendipitous Turn of Events

Jennifer was 91 with a shock of thick silver hair closely framing a face that had a healthy, sun-kissed glow about it. She walked into my office with a ready smile, accompanied by one of her daughters. Her usual moroseness and pallor had been wiped clean off her face, as if it had never existed. Amazingly, her memory had also improved. With a little help, Jennifer rattled off the names of the major political players and remembered what she had done a few weeks previously.

I was very surprised at this turn of events, for this was not the Jennifer I knew. Four years earlier, I had diagnosed her with slowly progressive Alzheimer's with excellent language skills, moderate memory loss, and mild life skill impairment. At the time,

Jennifer lived alone in a large suburban home but had become a recluse, her poor memory, depression, and pain from a bad knee all contributing to her isolation.

Her two devoted daughters and I saw Jennifer through a successful knee surgery and got her to accept a wonderful caregiver, Joan, who spent several hours each day with her, taking her out and making sure she took her medications. But even after her knee pain had resolved, and despite her amazing caregiver, Jennifer had remained depressed with an increasingly poor memory. Why the dramatic transformation now?

It turned out that the goddess of serendipity had been at work. Bonnie, a lifelong friend of Jennifer's, also widowed and living alone, was being discharged from a hospital after a protracted medical illness. Frail and 93, Bonnie was not quite strong enough to live alone, and Jennifer's daughters suggested that Bonnie spend time recuperating at their mother's home. Jennifer was happy to help an old friend and had plenty of room, and Joan, the caregiver, readily agreed to help if needed. Although physically frail, Bonnie had no cognitive issues. The arrangement was initially meant to be temporary, but it had suited all parties so well that it had become permanent. In the months since Bonnie had moved in, the two longtime friends settled into a comfortable, companionable routine.

"They have their coffee together outside on the deck, they listen to the birds, they take in the sun, and they never seem to run out of things to talk about," Jennifer's daughter marveled. "Joan has even started taking them hiking, and they just love it. It has been an all-round win-win situation."

Steeping in the tea of true companionship, Jennifer had lost her sense of despair and regained some of her memory. The unusual living arrangement worked not only for Jennifer and Bonnie, giving them dignity and freedom, but had allowed Joan, their caregiver, a woman in midlife, to find sustainable, meaningful employment. Jennifer's story gave me one more alternative to consider for others in similar situations.

Caregiving is a tough job, no matter how one looks at it, and one that family caregivers rarely envision as a part of their later years. Yet as we have seen, it can be fulfilling and uplifting in different ways, despite the enormous challenges and the changes it can cause in the primary relationship. Paid caregivers are a valuable part of the equation and should be welcomed into the mix when needed. Other family members, friends, and the community at large can help by offering support to the caregiver whenever possible. Finally, although living in one's own home is preferable for most, moving into a retirement facility or a nursing home may be a valid option for some patients on the spectrum.

CHAPTER 12
I THINK MY HUSBAND IS CHEATING ON ME WITH MY AIDE. NAVIGATING SEXUALITY: SUSPICION, AFFAIRS, AND SPECIAL ARRANGEMENTS

"How can I have sex with him?" the 72-year-old wife of a patient with Alzheimer's recently asked me. "I bathe and dress him like he is a baby. He seems like my child at this point. Sometimes we lie next to each other and he fondles my breasts, and that's comforting. But I can't imagine it going further than that anymore."

Caring for a spouse with dementia poses special challenges, as it alters the romantic landscape on which the relationship was based. Spouse caregivers may find themselves in the position of helping their romantic partners with toileting, bathing, and other very private activities. They may find that they have lost their dinner companion, their dance partner, the person who laughed at their jokes or made jokes, the person who helped them deal with life's curveballs.

Many spouses find it hard to maintain physical intimacy and a romantic relationship with the person they are also bathing and dressing.

Although being a caregiver for anyone with a chronic illness presents a number of challenges, taking care of loved ones with dementia can be especially difficult. If the patient denies the illness, they may not acknowledge or thank the caregiver for their efforts. Some patients may not be emotionally or cognitively available to meet the caregiver's sexual or romantic needs. Finally, of all the different family members who may pitch in and help, spouses spend the most amount of time with caregiving responsibilities and often risk depleting their emotional reserves.

As we've seen in earlier chapters, some spouse caregivers are able to adapt to these challenges and maintain strong physical and emotional bonds with their partners, despite the changed circumstances. Others find that they continue to love their spouses, but no longer in a romantic or sexual way.

Several articles in the last few years, in publications ranging from *The Wall Street Journal* to *AARP: The Magazine,* have addressed this issue. *AARP: The Magazine* recounted a story of a husband caregiver who became friendly with another woman — she became his dinner and movie companion — even as he continued to care for his wife. The article emphasized that the relationship was platonic — the husband did not cross the "line of decency."

In my practice, however, many caregivers of patients with Alzheimer's and other chronic illnesses have, in fact, crossed this so-called "line of decency." It may surprise you to learn that I do not judge these caregivers. Although I certainly do not advocate infidelity, I refuse to condemn excellent and loving caregivers who have sought to fulfill the basic human need for love and intimacy elsewhere when their partners are no longer able to provide it. In fact, the irony is that, in some cases, their transgression helps them to better care for their spouse with Alzheimer's.

ANNA'S STORY

Anna was a patient whose difficult life made me question whether inherent justice exists in the world. Despite being born and coming of age in war-torn Germany, Anna, in her sixties, maintained that curious mix of naïveté, dread, and conviction so characteristic of children. She had a penchant for rescuing abandoned baby squirrels in the park and nursing them back to health.

She lived through World War II, and although, as a Catholic, she wasn't directly persecuted by the Nazis, she nevertheless endured a tragic series of events. When she was 9 years old, her mother was placed in a sanitarium for tuberculosis. Anna saw her just once more, a year later, shortly before she died. An only child, Anna was left alone with her father, who happened to be a closeted homosexual — a group that was targeted by the Nazis. When Anna was about 13, her father was taken away and killed.

After his death, Anna was cared for by kind neighbors, because she had no other locatable relatives. At the age of 14, she was gang-raped on her way home from school, her first and only sexual experience until she was 21.

After this series of nightmarish events, Anna arrived in the United States at the age of 16 and was taken in by a family in Maryland. Unfortunately, because of lingering antiwar sentiment, she was vilified by many of her neighbors for being German. Further compounding her personal tragedy, Anna found herself unable to share the sad story of her life, having trouble finding a sympathetic shoulder to lean on.

Anna did not let her past deter her and went on to get a college degree. She met and married a man with whom she had two children. However, eight years into the marriage, she realized her beloved husband was cheating on her. After an acrimonious divorce, he left her without any support. Anna took on a series of jobs to support her two sons.

Eventually, she met and married Aaron, a man fifteen years younger, whom she rescued from the throes of alcoholism. Aaron's livelihood as a lawyer was being threatened by his drinking, and Anna single-handedly helped him conquer his addiction and achieve sobriety.

When I first met Anna, she was 62. She'd come to see me for help with long-term lower back pain, but she kept insisting that she was developing Alzheimer's. I put her through a series of tests and gave her my diagnosis: There was not a shred of evidence that she was developing the disease. Her memory seemed to be fine. In fact, she was actually one of the most brilliant people I had ever tested, attesting to her large level of cognitive reserve, which protected her from developing Alzheimer's.

Despite this, every three to four months when she came in about her back pain, she told me she knew she was developing Alzheimer's and that I was wrong.

"Anna, I know what I'm doing," I told her. "I've done an MRI, and I've checked your memory and cognition with a thorough evaluation. There is simply no sign that you're developing Alzheimer's.

"I think you may be depressed," I continued. "Perhaps the depression is making you feel vulnerable, like you're forgetting."

"I respect you, Doctor," Anna responded, "but I know myself, and I know my brain isn't working like it used to."

Over the course of these visits, I got to know Anna intimately. She told me the stories of her life, and we developed a close friendship within the construct of the doctor-patient relationship.

Every year she summered in Virginia Beach, and one September she came back to New York a completely changed woman. Her cognition was remarkably worse, and when I tested her, I discovered that Anna had indeed developed Alzheimer's disease. I had never seen a case like this where over the space of three months someone had deteriorated so rapidly. In the beginning, I was sure it was something else — an infection or cancerous process within the central nervous system or in the rest of the body, perhaps — but all the relevant tests, including a spinal tap, made the diagnosis clear. It was almost as if Anna had willed herself into developing Alzheimer's, although I knew that was impossible. I speculated that because she was so brilliant, Anna had compensated for the accumulating pathology in her brain by devising cognitive "work-arounds" until she was no longer able to cope and succumbed to the illness, which had already spread through much of her brain. She had done well in previous testing because of how smart she was.

Before she developed the disease, one of Anna's biggest fears was that Aaron would stray as her first husband had. Having been abandoned so often in her life, being left alone yet again was the thing she feared the most. By this time, her sons had grown up and were leading their own lives, so Aaron was her main source of social and emotional support.

Aaron continually reassured Anna that he would never betray her, both in my presence and in the privacy of their home. He told her repeatedly that she had saved his life, that he loved her with all his heart, and that he would stay faithful to her, and I believed the sincerity of his declarations.

The irony of this, as you may have already

guessed, is that he did end up betraying her, and in the most hurtful possible way. Anna progressed into a galloping dementia, the likes of which I've never seen before or since, and deteriorated rapidly. In the period of a year she went from being a vibrant, social, independent woman to someone with moderate to severe impairment of life skills, although her memory impairment was mild and her language skills were still good. Aaron had to hire around the clock caregivers to help her with bathing, dressing, and other activities. Yet even in the depths of her dementia, Anna was plagued by one fear: the possibility of her husband's infidelity.

One day, she came to see me, distraught. She told me that she had heard Aaron talking in his sleep. As he slept, he had repeatedly called out the name of one of Anna's caregivers, a young woman named Melanie.

"Dr. Devi, they're having an affair," Anna said.

When Anna confronted him, Aaron denied everything. "I don't talk in my sleep. Your dementia is making your mind play tricks on you."

This, of course, confused Anna greatly. She looked at me, her green eyes filled with tears, and said, "I don't know if it's true or not. Maybe I dreamed the whole thing. Tell me, Doctor, is my mind really playing tricks on me? Is it my dementia?"

"Anna," I replied, "let me talk to Aaron and find out."

THE DENOUEMENT

In my practice, I find it very helpful to meet with the patient and the caregiver — whether family or paid — together at the beginning of each visit. Then I meet briefly with the caregiver alone before spending the rest of my time with my patient. This helps me take better care of my patients, because I can advise each party about issues they may be reluctant to bring up in the presence of the other. For example, a caregiver may relate an episode of incontinence that they didn't want to embarrass the patient by bringing up, and a patient may complain about having "my life managed" without fear of offending the caregiver.

An additional benefit of these separate meetings with the caregiver is that they allow me to establish a relationship with them and help them find solutions for their daily struggles with the patient. If patients protest about being left out of my meetings with caregivers — and they sometimes do — I explain my position to them and emphasize that it helps me provide better care for them. Once they understand this, it is rare that they still complain.

Over the course of Anna's illness, Aaron and I had developed a good rapport, and after Anna told me her concerns privately, Aaron came in and confessed.

"I've gotten involved with Melanie," he admitted. "This is crazy to say, but after the hell of this last year with Anna, I have finally found some happiness. The thing is, Melanie's right there in the apartment, which makes it so convenient." Though Aaron sounded callous, he was still worried that Anna knew what was happening and was concerned about the effect it would have on her.

"I think Anna's gotten wind of it," he said. "I believe I talked about Melanie in my sleep and Anna heard me. I told her it was all a dream, but she doesn't believe me. You have to help me keep this lie going. It would destroy her if she knew. Anna is the best thing that ever happened to me. If it weren't for her, I would probably be dead in some gutter somewhere. I can't let her find out."

I was put in a terrible position. I was being asked to lie to my patient based on the risk of the emotional harm it would cause her, even as it felt almost physically repugnant to do so.

Anna's greatest fear was coming true, in the midst of her alarmingly rapidly progressive Alzheimer's. But had Aaron really abandoned her? He had not put her in a nursing home. He was helping to care for her in their own home, something that gave her great solace.

The decision I faced was this: Was I going to rupture the fragile world Aaron and Anna were living in by telling her the truth?

To this day I don't know if I did the right thing. I opted to collude with Aaron and tell Anna that it was all in her mind, that her husband loved her — which was true — and that as far as I could conclude, her husband and Melanie were not having a romantic relationship.

I remember Anna looking at me and saying, "Okay, then. If you say so, Doctor . . ."

I don't think she believed me. But I think she knew what I was trying to do and was forgiving me for it.

COMPASSION FOR THE CAREGIVER

You might wonder why I didn't resent Aaron for putting me in that situation. Honestly, I would rather he had told me than left me in the dark. I can make better-informed decisions and be more helpful when caregivers are frank with me, even about the darkest of things. I've dealt with many situations like Aaron's, whereas he was going through it for the very first time. In the reverse logic that guides some human behavior, straying caregivers like Aaron may take out their guilt by treating the patient more harshly, sometimes even to the point of violence. However, I have found that once they have "confessed" and don't feel judged, they are able to be kinder and gentler with their loved ones.

Why did Aaron take up with Melanie, his wife's aide, which seems particularly cruel? If he had to have an affair, why not pick someone farther from home? Based on other such situations, I don't think that the relationship arose from some special malice, but rather from the fact that Aaron and Melanie began to spend large amounts of time together caring for Anna and developed a bond that turned into a sexual dalliance. Would Aaron have been a better man if he had put his wife in a nursing home and not had an affair? From my perspective, no. Knowing Anna as I did, I think Aaron would have caused her far greater pain if he had put her in a facility that separated her from both her husband and her home.

Eight months into the affair, Anna broke her hip and died within a few weeks.

One may choose to vilify Aaron for his betrayal, but in some ways, strangely enough, I see Aaron as a hero because he chose to make and stick with a difficult decision. A deeply flawed hero and one I did not particularly care for, but a hero nonetheless. Aaron tried to do the best he could to satisfy everyone's needs, given the cards he was dealt. Not all of my patients have been so lucky in their choice of spouse.

ANOTHER TYPE OF BETRAYAL

Wendy was a very bright woman of 65 who taught architecture at one of the city's finest universities and came from a very wealthy family. She lived in a gorgeous brownstone with her husband, Dave, a fellow professor. They had met and married just five years earlier, and Wendy worshipped the ground he walked on.

Wendy had been referred to me by her longtime gynecologist, Sue, who was worried that Wendy was getting more forgetful. Wendy had failed to follow up on abnormal test results, having forgotten all about a long conversation they had had about them.

I was struck by Wendy's optimism the first time I met her. She told me how grateful she was for her life and that she had been very lucky. "The most delightful thing in my life," she said, "is my husband, Dave. He came to me magically, a prince on a white horse, late in my life when I had given up on meeting anyone, and he has given my life meaning. He is wonderful."

I tested Wendy and diagnosed her with rapidly progressive Alzheimer's disease, with mild language and memory loss and good life skills. Once Wendy and I had gone over the diagnosis and prognosis, as well as available treatment options, we decided that she would return to my office with her husband so that he could help her settle on a treatment regimen.

Upon meeting Dave, I was skeptical. I didn't like him much, but I couldn't put my finger on why. Wendy had initially been eager to begin treatment, but after the visit with Dave, she came back into my office and said brightly, "Dave says I'm fine. That maybe you and my gynecologist are overreacting. He says my memory is as good as his, and he has a great memory."

"But what do *you* think, Wendy?" I asked.

Sadly, she had already decided that there was not much wrong with her, which suited her natural optimism. When she came in for her checkups — which she did despite refusing to admit she had a problem — she remained chipper and positive and glowed whenever she spoke of "my Dave." As Wendy's illness progressed and she lost her job, Dave continued to deny her problems and steadfastly refused any kind of treatment for her. It was then that I realized that his motives were not altogether kosher.

When I spoke with Sue, Wendy's gynecologist, to see if she could persuade Wendy to agree to treatment, she concurred with my impressions of Dave.

"I've had a hard time not being suspicious of Dave," Sue confessed. She was a bit of a mother hen with many of her patients, taking an interest in all aspects of their life. "I have known Wendy since she was 21; she became a patient just after I started my practice. She was so excited to meet Dave — she thought she would never get hitched. I gathered there may have been some pressure from his end for their getting married, and I told her to make sure to sign a prenup. Wendy told me there was no need, that she'd spoken to him and he'd told her it would not be 'true love' if they did."

Even as Wendy got worse and worse, she continually praised her husband. Every time they were in the office together, Dave would be very solicitous of her, fawning over her like she was a queen. She would melt over these expressions of affection. But the minute she left the room and Dave and I were alone, a visible change would come over him. He would become practical — even coldhearted. He would talk about his need to put her away. He spoke about how she was cramping his lifestyle. He complained that he hadn't planned on being married to a woman who was going to get ill so quickly after their wedding. Dave made it very clear to me that he really had no interest in maintaining Wendy's quality of life. He felt no need to keep up any pretense with me, because the two of us had already argued about the fact that Wendy wasn't on any medication. When he was with Wendy, he was an actor and she was his captive audience, but I was not important. I believe he allowed her to continue to see me only to cast himself as a valiant detractor to my claims that she was ill and needed medical help.

Despite my entreaties, Dave would not consider in-home care, so Wendy ended up in a nursing home. Her husband ended up with her brownstone. I no longer saw or was able to keep in touch with Wendy after she was placed in the nursing facility. For her sake, I hope she went to her grave still believing she had married her prince, the man who loved her above all else.

THREE'S COMPANY

In at least a dozen other cases, I've been visited by a patient, her husband, and his mistress all at once. The mistress is frequently a friend, someone who works with the husband, or someone who is involved in the care of the patient. Oddly, the trio often becomes a happy family, and if not happy, then at least comfortable. I am not sure whether my patients are conscious of the affair going on in front of them, but I can't imagine that they aren't at least a little aware. I rarely probe further into these situations, because they are best left alone in most cases.

Family members of such "straying" caregivers, however, may have a tough time dealing with these arrangements.

Lola, an architect friend, told me the story of her parents, who were happily married for thirty-five years until, in her sixties, her mother had a series of small strokes. Each stroke left her more debilitated, to the point where she was no longer able to move. She also developed a vascular dementia from the multiple strokes. Lola and her father arranged for in-home care.

400

"I was visiting my mum," Lola told me. "Dorothy, an old friend from my parents' college days, stopped by. My mother didn't greet her warmly, which was puzzling, because Dorothy seemed very nice. I hadn't seen Dorothy since I was a child, and I didn't understand what Mum had against her. Mum could barely communicate, but I tried to get her to tell me why she didn't like this woman. She finally got through to me that Dorothy was my dad's mistress.

"At first I was angry with Dorothy and furious with my dad. I couldn't bring myself to speak to him for days, I was so beside myself. But once I calmed down, I stopped and said to myself, *I know my dad loves my mum, I know she loves him too, and I know that they can't have sex because she's too ill.* Then it occurred to me that perhaps having another person involved in his life helped my dad be a better caregiver.

"I think I'm learning to think like you, Gayatri!" Lola continued. "All your talks about caregivers must be rubbing off. I wondered if I was being selfish by expecting him to remain celibate through all this."

When Lola changed her perspective, she came to understand her father's bind, and, funnily enough, also came to appreciate his mistress.

"Eventually my mum came to accept and, I think, even love Dorothy a little. In some ways, Dorothy was probably better with my mum than I ever was," Lola confessed. "Some people may think it was creepy, but she was a saint. She helped bathe my mum and changed her diapers."

Now that her mother is gone, Lola is happy that her father has a companion in Dorothy. She says that both she and her father feel closer to this woman, who stood by and supported him through some of the most trying times of his life. Not only that, but they both value that Dorothy knew and cared about Lola's mother.

FEMALE CAREGIVERS

In my experience, women assume caregiving responsibilities more readily, with less protest and more resignation than men. Perhaps as a result, women suffer more from depression and anxiety than their male counterparts. And in contrast to male caregivers, few female caregivers I've met in my practice opt to seek physical solace outside the marriage, choosing instead to remain without intimacy.

As with most generalizations, there are exceptions. Samantha was the 44-year-old attractive and caring wife of my patient

Barney, who was diagnosed with rapidly progressive Alzheimer's at age 56. He died six years later, bed bound for the last year of his life. Samantha initially cared for him on her own, in addition to tending to their young children.

About two years into Barney's illness, the day-to-day care became too much for Samantha to handle on her own. Together, she, Barney, and I decided it was time to hire a live-in aide. We settled on a man because Barney said he would be more comfortable with one and because we needed someone strong enough to lift him when necessary.

Phil, the aide, was just the person for Barney and Samantha. He was a fit 40-year-old with experience caring for patients with dementia. He and Barney hit it off immediately and would go for long walks together as long as Barney was able. They watched football games on television. Samantha and Barney's two teenage children got used to seeing Phil around the house.

About three years into his dementia, a year after Phil had joined them, Barney told me, "I am happy we have Phil around. Sam has such a job on her hands with me and the kids."

"Nonsense!" Samantha said. "We love you

and that's that. I don't want to hear that type of talk."

Less than two years after this conversation, Barney became mute and had trouble recognizing his family. He moved out of the marital bedroom because of his incontinence and now shared the guest room with Phil.

Around this time, things took an unexpected turn.

"We are falling in love, Phil and I," Samantha blurted one afternoon when we were talking in my office, her eyes full of tears. "I love Barney, you know I do. But when we are changing him, or showering him together, it's as if Phil and I are parents caring for our sick child."

Samantha and Phil kept their relationship secret for nearly a year after Phil's death, but they eventually married. Samantha kept in touch with me by telephone. She told me that she had moved to Colorado with Phil and her children because both her family and Barney's disapproved of her actions. Barney's mother and sister had gone so far as to call Samantha a whore, she said.

"How are the kids doing?" I asked.

"They love Phil," she said. "He's been like a second father to them. I just wish our families would understand. I never meant to do this, but don't I deserve some happiness? I know Barney would understand and want this for me."

This was the only instance in my practice where I became aware of the wife of a patient becoming involved sexually with another man, but surely there are other cases. I believe, in any event, that such painful and clearly conflicted decisions made by loving caregivers, whether men or women, deserve support, not opprobrium.

SEXUAL ANTICS

Sometimes, it is the patient with dementia who becomes more sexually adventurous as the illness progresses, often to the consternation of the caregiver.

Early in my career, at the age of 28, back when I found it difficult to believe that anyone over the age of 60 actually had sex, I had a patient with Alzheimer's named John who was in his eighties. One afternoon, his wife, Marie, also in her eighties, came to see me. She had rosy cheeks and curly, white hair, with exposed bits of baby-pink scalp between strands. Marie was generally quite reserved.

"You have to help me with a new problem, Doctor," she declared. "John is getting very randy."

"What do you mean?" I asked.

"Well, the other evening, when our whole family was over for dinner — everyone sitting around the kitchen table — John tried to have sex with me as I was trying to get something out of the oven!"

John was exhibiting some of the behavioral disinhibition and lapses in judgment that occur with some patients on the Alzheimer's spectrum. The ability to maintain control of one's impulses and make socially appropriate decisions is the province of our frontal lobes, but when this area is affected by dementia, our judgment suffers. Such disinhibition occurs particularly often in patients with frontotemporal dementia, whose frontal lobes are invariably affected. Sometimes issues like John's can be helped by medication, but redirection is likely to be more effective.

Another patient of mine, Dan, exhibited a subtler form of judgment lapse. Eighty-six years old, he was a charming man with tanned skin and a square jaw with a dimple in the middle, like Clark Gable's. Despite his advanced age, he had a full head of lustrous silver hair that he wore swept to one side. He had slowly progressive Alzheimer's with mild memory loss and intact language and life skills. He was functional, still working at his job as a senior executive at a major media firm, although he had become more irritable at work.

Known for his gentle temperament, he had started to become argumentative. I attributed his behavior change partly to his Alzheimer's and partly to the fact that he was now the part-time caregiver of his wife, who was in the end stages of cancer. I placed him on a small dose of an anti-depressant to curb his irritability, which was helpful. However, he shocked me at a visit a few months later when he began to complain about his wife's colostomy bag.

"It's hard to get turned on by a woman who's dying," Dan told me bluntly. "I'd like to have sex, but I can't because she doesn't seem that into it."

"Dan," I said, shocked and showing it, "of course she's not into it — you don't seem to understand how ill she is."

"I know she's sick," he said, waving away my disbelief, "but I can't help my needs. Not to mention, the colostomy bag is a real turnoff."

Although I was appalled by Dan's callousness with regard to his wife's plight, I tried to understand things from his perspective and not be too harsh in judging him. I knew that Dan loved his wife, and I knew his Alzheimer's disease had interfered with his impulse control. He was also responding to a loss of intimacy, although in a manner that was difficult to hear. There was nothing I could do to help Dan with his dilemma.

A LOVE STORY

Thankfully, not all of the stories of my patients' romantic lives push the envelope of what constitutes the definition of "acceptable" behavior. It's rare, but some scripts for "new" lives can have universal appeal with a happily-ever-after ending.

Beverley developed mildly progressive Alzheimer's at 70. A warm, kind woman, Beverley had been blissfully married to Jack for more than a half century, and she was prone to dispensing advice. I remember her standing on the scale in my office one morning and handing me a life pearl to live by.

"Don't wait until you retire to have fun, to go on vacation," she said. "Look at Jack and me — we were busy raising our children, so we kept putting things off for when we got older. Now here I am, sick! Make sure you have fun every day."

I was 31 when she told me this, but something in her gravity and sincerity as she spoke made a deep impression on me. I took her advice to heart and have followed it ever since. I make sure to schedule daily and weekly downtimes and have been fiercely and unapologetically protective of my "me time." I am positive that this "me time" has made me a better, more patient physician. I try to impart Beverley's lessons to my patients and their caregivers as well.

I treated Beverley aggressively, with a combination of approved medication and cognitive therapy. Along the way, Beverley also had surgery to drain the excess fluid in her brain, a condition known as hydrocephalus. She was stable for more than ten years before progressing and dying at 82.

Jack was just as effusive and friendly as Beverley and cared for her tenderly until the very end. Three years after her death, he showed up at my office for an impromptu visit. Although he had moved to Florida, he would drop by unannounced whenever he was in New York City. I welcomed his surprise visits, because they reminded me of our years caring for Beverley together and of the love they shared.

This time, Jack had brought a visitor, Camilla. Camilla had been the maid of honor at Jack and Beverley's wedding, and her husband had been the best man, just as Beverley and Jack had been the maid of honor and best man at Camilla's wedding. Now Camilla's husband had died, and Camilla and Jack had gotten together.

"Camilla," Jack said, introducing us, "meet the doctor who took care of Beverley."

I was moved to tears. I felt honored to continue being a part of Beverley's life even after she was gone. To this day, every January, I receive a box of sunny Florida oranges from Jack, who must be nearing 90, and it brings warmth into my life.

LOVE IN THE TIME OF DEMENTIA

Some couples continue to enjoy sexual or affectionate physical relationships with each other even when one partner has dementia. Dolores and Adam were a lovely couple, both in their eighties, and Dolores had slowly progressive Alzheimer's.

"Dolores and I have always enjoyed a wonderful and close physical relationship," Adam said about their sex life. "The funny thing is, now that she has Alzheimer's, we've become even closer. We love to be together, and I think we both enjoy it as much now, if not more."

"Yes," Dolores said, nodding in agreement. "I love being with Adam. It's wonderful when we are together."

Dolores went through some challenging phases in her illness, at one point becoming convinced that Adam was stealing from her. We were able to successfully treat these and other symptoms with medication. Dolores and Adam continued to stay close, both emotionally and physically. I think it helped that Adam hired a caregiver, a wonderful woman who was attuned to Dolores and helped her with her daily activities, which allowed Adam to continue to see Dolores as his romantic beloved rather than as his charge.

Ali and Bart are another example of love thriving in spite of dementia. Ali, 82, had slowly progressive Alzheimer's with moderate-severe memory loss and excellent verbal and life skills. Bart, who doted on Ali, was scruffily handsome at 83, and they made a striking pair. They laughed constantly, as I suspect they had done throughout their sixty-plus years of marriage.

Ali had recently begun to see many versions of Bart. She was suffering from Capgras syndrome, where a person thinks a familiar person has been replaced by an exact duplicate, an uncommon and particularly disconcerting delusion seen in some patients on the spectrum. When a spouse is thought to be an imposter, there is tremendous anxiety and bewilderment not only for the patient but also for the caregiver. Imagine waking up in bed next to a stranger, or imagine being awakened and treated like a stranger by your wife of fifty-odd years. Bart, however, was taking it in stride.

"It is an interesting challenge to not get upset about it and try to get her to understand that there is only one of me. . . . She understands, but a part of her keeps the other thread going. Last week Ali was seeing too many versions of me for too much of the week. . . ."

Both Ali and Bart burst into laughter at this.

"She asks me, 'Where did he go?' meaning where did I go," Bart continued.

"Is this true, Ali?" I asked her.

"I don't recall," Ali said. "But it is funny!"

"We were sitting and having breakfast yesterday," Bart said. "And Ali said to me, 'I wonder if he's coming back — he made a great dinner last night.' I told her I was the one who made the dinner. Even though I can get her to agree that there is just one person, the next sentence she goes back to asking where 'he' is. Sometimes, I do get upset. But mostly, I have learned to live with it."

"He's just making this stuff up," Ali said,

after listening carefully to Bart. "He's talking about my delusion. It's not a delusion, it's a point of view."

"I have to learn to be less rigid in my definitions," Bart agreed. "I have to be comfortable being 'he' and me at the same time."

Unfortunately, there was nothing I could do about Ali's Capgras syndrome. I couldn't talk Ali out of her intermittent but firmly held belief that her husband was a duplicate, delusional as it was. Sometimes, medications used for anxiety and agitation can help when the delusion results in severe distress, but Bart and Ali were doing well enough on their own, so I opted not to monitor or treat it.

Bart and Ali also talked to me about sexuality.

"We like to snuggle," Bart said. "I can't perform sexually anymore, but I get so lecherous, it's hard to handle."

"Up to a point it's nice," Ali said with a smile. "Then I push him away."

They sauntered jauntily out of my office together, one guiding the other, and I thought, *Love is a many splendored thing.*

Caregiving is a difficult, draining task, and there can be a breathtaking loneliness to it. Spouse caregivers may opt to choose the solace of physical intimacy in ways that may be frowned upon by society. Interestingly, because of the rising incidence of such arrangements, some religious leaders have gone so far as to think about a redefinition of the term *adultery* in these circumstances. Having repeatedly witnessed it up close over many years, and with the most loving of couples, I now understand why it happens and have learned to not be critical of it.

Some spouse caregivers, like Bart, find ways to make peace with the new "normal," finding joy and fulfillment in loving and caring for their spouse or partner, who now has an illness that changes their relationship in irrevocable ways. Regardless of what form it takes, I strive to always understand and appreciate the spouse-caregiver relationship and be as supportive as possible.

CHAPTER 13
SHOULD I GO TO THE HOSPITAL IF I'M SICK?
TREATING MEDICAL ILLNESS ALONGSIDE DEMENTIA

In my experience, patients with Alzheimer's who have other medical illnesses are best treated at home rather than in a hospital. The disorienting unfamiliarity of the hospital, the muscle-atrophying enforced bed rests, and busy personnel not attuned to the specific needs of the patient all contribute to less-than-optimal conditions for recovery. For these reasons, I prefer home-based care.

Conditions that commonly lead to patients with dementia being hospitalized include dizziness, urinary tract infections, pneumonias, and falls, all of which can be successfully and more comfortably treated at home. Some of these medical illnesses can exhibit themselves as increasing confusion in patients with dementia and can puzzle caregivers, who don't know what's causing the change. Surprisingly, hip fractures may also be either treated or rehabilitated at home. Depending on the fracture type, up to a third of such fractures can be treated with just bed rest, pain management, and physical therapy.

Of course, the patient's internist needs to be supportive of a home-based approach, which places a greater burden of medical oversight on the physician. However, when feasible, I strongly recommend home-based care, because I have consistently found it to be the best route to a good outcome for my patients on the spectrum.

URINARY TRACT INFECTIONS

Andy was a 78-year-old retired engineer, tall and thin, with Lewy body dementia. Symptoms in this condition can resemble Parkinson's, and, in fact, there is some degree of overlap between the two. Andy moved in slow motion, and his strong voice had faded to a whisper.

"Speak up, Andy!" his wife, Sabra, would frequently plead during their visits to my office. "Speak up, for heaven's sake! We can't hear you!"

As his movements slowed, Andy became more and more confined to their apartment he became markedly stooped, his reedy frame nearly draped over itself. Sabra, a tiny woman, valiantly pushed and pulled him along, but after a while, his physical care became too much for her. Even so, she was determined to keep him at home, a sentiment more often expressed by female caregivers than male. After much resistance from Sabra — I felt like I was pulling teeth — she reluctantly agreed to get a part-time paid caregiver. This kind of resistance from a caregiver is far more usual than the ready acceptance of necessary help.

As his illness progressed, we changed Andy's medications to best help his many symptoms, including memory loss, depression, and slowed mobility. Patients with Lewy body dementia are particularly sensitive to medication and may react very strongly, suffering serious side effects if they are not closely monitored. After yet another medication change, Andy suddenly became very confused. Sabra called me one morning.

"Andy is delirious," she said. "He's talking nonsense; it's been nothing but gibberish for two days straight. I try to talk to him, but he gazes past me with a vacant look in his eyes. Last night, he started hallucinating, and this morning he was tearing off his sheets. When I asked him why, he told me that little bugs were running up and down his bed. I think I should take him to the emergency room."

"Bring him here to the office," I said. "The hospital may just confuse him even further."

When he came in, helped by his aide and his wife, Andy seemed calm and was co-operative with my questions. Although he was somewhat drowsy, he did not have a temperature. I suspected he was having a reaction to the new medication, so I stopped it just to be safe. Visual hallucinations can be a symptom of Lewy body dementia, but the onset seemed too sudden for that to be the cause.

Medical illnesses can manifest themselves in unusual ways in patients with dementia, so after I finished his exam — which showed no evidence of an infection — I obtained samples of his blood and urine for testing just in case. The evaluation revealed that Andy had, in fact, developed a urinary tract infection. This was the culprit in his altered mental state. Patients with dementia are more likely than the rest of us to develop confusion from the metabolic changes caused by infection. Putting Andy on an oral antibiotic to treat the infection resolved the problem, and he returned to his baseline within a week. Despite symptoms sugges-tive of a dramatic worsening of his demen-tia, Andy's condition turned out to be an easily treated infection and was well managed at home.

Medical illness can dramatically exacerbate the symptoms of dementia. Patients who have experienced falls or infections may suddenly lose the ability to control their bowels or bladder. Others, like Andy, may also suddenly lose the ability to speak coherently, which understandably alarms their families, who are expecting a gradual change in cognition, not a precipitous decline. It's important to reassure families that once the illness is treated, the patient should return to their baseline, though it can sometimes take as long as a few months for recovery.

As I mentioned, whenever possible, I try to manage illness at home, even when other physicians would advocate hospitalization. The unfamiliarity of a disorienting new environment, with rigid routines and unfamiliar staff, can exacerbate anxiety and agitation. Patients may try to get out of bed on their own, putting them at risk for falls and fractures. Patients may be given medication to calm them down, and those have their own side effects, including sedation and drowsiness. They may have difficulty communicating with unfamiliar caregivers, further increasing agitation. For example, an unfamiliar nurse may fail to pick up on a patient-specific signal for bathroom use.

Additionally, hospitals, by their very nature, require patients to be in bed for much of the day. In one study, hospitals allowed patients out of bed for a mere forty-three minutes each day. As a result, elderly hospitalized patients can lose up to 10 percent of the lean muscle mass in their legs in as little as three days. When compounded by the fact that patients with dementia have longer average hospital stays than their peers without dementia, the case for home-based medical management becomes stronger. I can personally recollect numerous cases when I was unable to prevent hospitalization, either because the family or the patient's internist objected, and my patients left hospitals in a wheelchair after walking in. It is important to appreciate that patients without dementia have more positive hospital experiences than those with dementia.

TREATING PNEUMONIA AT HOME

My 74-year-old patient Kathleen took much longer to recover from her pneumonia than Andy did from his urinary tract infection. She had been living alone in her house in Long Island, stable with her Alzheimer's, when she developed severe pneumonia. The symptoms were compounded by her forty-year history of smoking two packs a day. Kathleen suddenly became incontinent, could no longer drive, and had trouble dialing the phone. Within a matter of days, she went from having a life of her own to needing constant oversight and help from her daughter Tina.

Once I diagnosed her pneumonia, we treated her at home with a powerful oral antibiotic, and a chest X-ray a week later showed that the pneumonia had largely resolved. Even so, she remained confused and did not immediately recover her continence.

Tina, who was raising two young children, was alarmed by the persistent change in her mother.

"You told me this was all from the pneumonia, but it's been two weeks since she finished her treatment, and she's still not back to normal," she said. "Mom's still not making sense — in fact, she's now getting lost inside the house — and she's still wetting the bed. I can't be there all the time. Do we need to put her in a home?"

"You've got to give it time," I told her. "Please give it another week or two. I promise she will slowly come back to normal."

Sure enough, in about a month Kathleen was back to her old self, managing on her own, no longer getting lost, no longer incontinent, and back to her two-pack-a-day habit. Educating Tina about the time Kathleen needed to recover was helpful in reducing her anxiety about her mother and helped keep Kathleen at home, where she wanted to be.

THE RUSH TO TREAT

Sometimes when a patient appears ill, anxious family members insist on "doing something!" even if it leads to needless, and possibly harmful, intervention. In such situations, the availability of multiple medical opinions, with varying recommendations, can aggravate the situation.

I once got a call early in the morning from the son of my patient Victoria, telling me that his mother had become more confused overnight.

"Mom doesn't seem like herself," he told me. "She looks groggy and is more disoriented than usual."

"Is she complaining of pain anywhere?" I asked.

"No," he said. "She just seems confused."

"Let's wait and see how the day progresses," I said. In patients with dementia, some fluctuation in level of alertness is normal — it's unrelated to infections or other external causes, and often resolves on its own. I knew the increased confusion could be a transient, benign fluctuation in the symptoms of Victoria's dementia. Her son reluctantly agreed to wait.

However, in quick succession, I received calls from both of Victoria's daughters, followed by one from the elder daughter's internist — who had never met Victoria — all telling me the same thing: Victoria needed immediate treatment.

I still counseled them to give it a little more time, to wait and see. However, the family was very concerned about their mother's recent change in mental status, and the idea of inaction felt positively scandalous to them.

Victoria's son succeeded in getting a doctor friend to visit his mother. The friend, a cardiologist, thought that Victoria might be suffering from a urinary tract infection and suggested that she go on antibiotics. One of the daughters called to fill me in.

"But how does she seem?" I asked.

"A little better than this morning," the daughter confessed, "but she's still confused."

"Why don't we try to get a sample of her

urine," I suggested, "and send it to be tested before we treat her? We should have the results in a few hours, and she can wait that long, particularly if she seems better."

Victoria's daughter agreed to collect a urine sample and drop it off at the local lab but persisted, along with her siblings, in asking for treatment for a presumed infection. No one was satisfied until I called in a prescription for antibiotics. Although treating with antibiotics pending laboratory results is acceptable care, I was sure that Victoria's diminishing confusion signified that an infection was nonexistent.

This knee-jerk reflex to resort quickly to antibiotics, even in cases where they are not indicated, such as viral sniffles and even the flu, is one of my problems with modern medicine. Antibiotics are particularly overused in the elderly, and if a patient develops resistance, they end up needing more powerful and more difficult-to-tolerate drugs. I refrain from using antibiotics unless there is a clear indication of bacterial infection, because my patients with dementia often respond poorly to them. They may develop side effects such as nausea, diarrhea, and agitation, which in turn can cause dehydration, low blood pressure, and more confusion, possibly leading to falls and fractures as they try to climb out of bed or walk out of their hospital room.

It was with great unwillingness that I started Victoria on antibiotics. A few hours later, her urine tests came back negative, and the family agreed to stop treatment. Even so, Victoria had been exposed unnecessarily to a drug she did not need. Fortunately, however, she was back to her usual self by the next morning.

The following weekend, I got another call from Victoria's daughter. "Mom developed a cough on Friday," she said. "We took her to the local urgent care center. They did an X-ray and think she has pneumonia, so now she's at the hospital emergency room."

"Whatever you do," I told her, "do not allow your mother to be admitted to the hospital. Please wait for the results of the X-rays to be officially read."

Chastened from our experience the week before, she waited, and sure enough, Victoria was cleared for discharge. What had been mistaken for pneumonia on Victoria's initial X-ray was found, on the final reading, to be no more than the distant scar of treated tuberculosis from her Eastern European childhood.

Victoria returned home safe and sound, without any long-term consequences. Another patient may not have been as lucky. Although waiting may be hard when a loved one is not doing well, sometimes, as in Victoria's case, it is the best thing to do. I am glad that I was able to prevent her from being hospitalized. Had she been admitted and "worked up," she would have been further disoriented. The numerous tests and procedures would have aggravated her confusion. She may have, in the interim, been placed on stronger antibiotics in the hospital, which may have caused side effects. Alternatively, she could have picked up a virulent hospital infection during her stay. In my experience, many patients on the spectrum who get admitted to hospitals stay an average four to five days, become more physically frail, and are more prone to falls and fractures upon their release.

A Cautionary Tale

Although we may think of antibiotics as a relatively benign treatment that's "no big deal," they can have devastating effects on the elderly. My friend Sandy told me the story of her aunt, who, at 103, was living in her own home and still had "all her marbles." However, she had outlasted her pacemaker, which had been placed in her chest wall many years before. Although it was still functioning, it was "coming out of her skin" and needed replacement. Given the skin breakdown, her aunt was prescribed what Sandy described as "some really strong antibiotics" as a way to prevent infection before the new pacemaker was inserted.

"When I went to see her, she was completely knocked out by this medication," Sandy said. "I called the doctor and he said to keep her on it. But by the end of the week, my aunt had stopped eating, she couldn't speak, and she was pooping and peeing on herself. It got so bad, I ended up calling emergency, and they put her in the hospital. I didn't know whether she would make it. At one point, she literally saw God and told him, 'Go back! Go back!' "

After the new pacemaker was put in, Sandy's aunt was eventually discharged to go home. "Truthfully," Sandy said, "after that, she was never the same again. She's a hundred and six now, and she'd still be kicking ass if it weren't for that medicine. As it is, she has had full-time care since two days after we started that antibiotic."

Pneumonia in the Hospital

Stella was 88 when she came to see me. She had Lewy body dementia, but had been misdiagnosed with Parkinson's disease — which can sometimes be difficult to differentiate from Lewy body dementia — and placed on medications for it. These medications made her simultaneously drowsy and agitated. To calm her down, she was given other medications, which made her more rigid and immobile, resulting in a large bedsore in the middle of her bent spine. For the pain resulting from the sore, Stella was put on narcotic medication, which made her even more drowsy and agitated.

When I first met Stella, she was in a wheelchair and barely awake. She was a slender woman, hunched over and held in place by her wheelchair straps, a sharp contrast to her tall and hearty husband of 90. They had been married for sixty-plus years and she had had round-the-clock help at home for a few years. Her husband made all of her medical decisions for her, because Stella was not able to do so.

Over a period of several weeks, with her husband's consent, I slowly reduced and then stopped her Parkinson's medication, and she became more alert. A wound specialist was found to visit her at home to care for her bedsore, which healed over three months. At that point, I was able to gradually decrease and then stop her narcotic medication, which she had been taking for her bedsore pain. Her mobility improved, and once I put her on medications for her dementia, she started to smile and even crack a joke or two.

Although Stella was never completely oriented or able to carry on an extended conversation, her quality of life improved dramatically. She regained the ability to stand, and walked with assistance for at least a half hour a day.

"How are you feeling, Stella?" I would ask when she visited.

"Good!" she would say with a smile, which delighted me.

However, Stella's story did not end well. Unfortunately, she developed pneumonia, with labored breathing and progressive drowsiness. Despite my protestations, her internist, a well-intentioned young man who had recently graduated from residency, insisted on hospitalizing her. I advocated for Stella to be treated with medication at home; he argued that Stella seemed medically unstable.

"Yes," I said, "but I'm not sure that a hospital stay would necessarily improve her quality of life, even if she were safely discharged."

Stella's husband, cautious by nature and worried about his wife, thought it was prudent to go the "safe" route.

Although her internist initially had estimated a three- or four-day stay, Stella was in the hospital for nine days. Two days after arriving, she developed a urinary tract infection from the catheter that had been placed into her bladder upon admission, a routine procedure for inpatients like Stella, even when they are continent. Already on antibiotics for her pneumonia, the additional infection, a virulent one, meant that she was switched to a different, stronger intravenous antibiotic.

She also spent a short time in the cardiac care unit because she developed heart problems. She endured multiple blood draws every day, and her arms and hands became a patchwork of splotches and bruises. She was seen by several consultants for all of her various problems, including a physiatrist for her mobility, an infectious diseases consultant, and a cardiologist. Disoriented and sedated on multiple medications, Stella stopped sitting up in bed. A speech and swallowing evaluation found that she was having trouble swallowing, and she had a nasogastric tube placed. Stella underwent many other diagnostic tests, not comprehending what they were. She had to be sedated for these tests, because she could not cooperate.

When I saw Stella in the hospital, I wanted to weep in sadness and outrage. She lay on her back — which was the most painful position she could be in, given the bedsore in the middle of her spine, which had reopened and was flourishing because of her immobility — in a hospital bed with all its sides up to prevent falls. She had the obligatory intravenous lines going in and out.

For what purpose? I remember fuming, angry with all of us physicians in general. *Why are we putting Stella through this?*

By the time of her discharge, Stella had lost several pounds from her already frail frame, despite her feeding tube. She had lost her recently regained ability to stand. She returned home in a wheelchair, hospice was called, and she died a week later. I firmly believe that had we treated Stella's pneumonia at home, she would have had a much better chance of a full recovery. Although there was a chance that she would have died sooner with the less aggressive treatment, she would have done so without all the suffering she endured in the hospital.

In the stories so far, the diagnosis was an infection of some sort that clearly would have been best treated at home. But what if the diagnosis is something like a hip fracture, where hospitalization seems like the only option?

TREATING A HIP FRACTURE AT HOME

One afternoon, I got a call from Nancy, the daughter of my patient Debbie, who was a slight, determined woman of 88 with Alzheimer's. She had been diagnosed nearly six years earlier and still lived alone in a small one-bedroom apartment. Over the last year, she'd had an aide with her several days a week to assist with shopping and other chores.

"My mom fell, and I think she broke her hip," Nancy told me. "She's screaming in pain and I don't know what to do." Nancy had called me instead of dialing 911 because in conversations over the years, we'd agreed to treat her mom's illnesses at home.

"Nancy," I replied, "if we take her to the hospital, I'm sure her hip will get fixed, but as you know, I think your mom is going to have a difficult time there. She likely won't be able to cooperate with the rehabilitation.

Is that what you'd like to do, or would you prefer that I manage her at home?"

"I'd prefer that Mom stay at home," she said. "It's what she wanted and what I want."

"You understand that her fracture may go unfixed?" I asked.

"Yes, I understand that," Nancy replied, "but I don't want her to go through all the trauma of being in a hospital."

"Do you understand that by keeping Debbie at home, we're allowing for the possibility that she might die?"

"Yes," Nancy said. "I'm very aware of that, but Mom has been adamant about staying away from hospitals, and I want to respect her wishes."

With this directive, Nancy, Debbie's aide, and I charted a course of action. I prescribed morphine to help manage Debbie's pain, and gave Nancy directions on how to administer the liquid. We contacted a visiting nurse agency to help Nancy and the aide with it. Nancy also hired another aide so that help was available at all hours of the day and night. As soon as my schedule allowed later that day, I went to see Debbie and found her asleep, resting from the morphine. I examined her, and what I found was consistent with a diagnosis of a hip fracture, although I could confirm the diagnosis only by X-ray. Under the circumstances, there was no point in getting X-rays.

Over the next few days, we gave Debbie morphine when she needed it for pain, and she began to slowly sit up in bed and eat. She was in bed for almost a week and then began to get up and move around, at which point, I arranged for a physical therapist to visit her in her home.

Debbie not only survived the hip fracture, but healed and started walking again, using a walker. She continued to visit me in my office for a few more years until she died at home.

When Nancy and I discussed this period of Debbie's life, neither of us had any regrets. The fact that Debbie survived and did well was icing on the cake, but both Nancy and I agreed that even if Debbie had not survived the fracture and had died at home, we had still made the right decision.

A third to a half of all hip fractures can be treated this way, and it may be an option to consider for an elderly patient with dementia who may not do well with hospitalization, surgery, and rehabilitation. Of course, other factors need to be weighed as well, including the difficulty of keeping a patient with dementia at home in bed, the risk for blood clots, and the very significant need for at-home help to allow this to happen.

A HOMETOWN CELEBRITY

A similar series of events occurred with Tina, a tiny, frail 90-year-old widow who had been living with her 85-year-old sister for many years. Tina had been diagnosed with slowly progressive Alzheimer's five years earlier, and had mild memory and life skills impairment and excellent language skills. For the last year she had had an aide help her for a few hours a day at home, but even so, she was still walking and went to work three days a week at her family's clothing store, charming customers into impulse buys with her astute salesmanship.

One afternoon, however, she fell and broke her hip, requiring surgery. Tina was the matriarch of a large and involved family — she had eight children and four surviving siblings — and at least twelve people were making decisions about her care. Her children and siblings and their spouses and children all crowded into the hospital, all wanting to be involved in the process.

After the operation, despite my counsel to take her home, the family decided to transfer her to an inpatient rehabilitation facility.

Once there, Tina refused to participate in her own rehabilitation. She would not get out of bed, moaned in pain, and was given narcotic medication every few hours. By the end of a week, it was clear that she was dying. She wasn't eating or drinking, and she barely acknowledged the numerous family members milling around her. Once I saw the state she was in, I knew I had to convince them to take her home.

"If she's going to die, why don't we let her die at home?" I told the family.

After much raucous discussion, Tina's family agreed to take her home to spend her last days. I told them the likelihood was high that Tina would be dead within a few days. However, once Tina got home, she rapidly perked up. She went from barely moving to recovering her appetite and mobility. She began to willingly participate in physical therapy.

I made visits to her home until she recuperated enough to visit me at my office. I enjoy visiting my patients on their own turf because there's a power shift. When a patient comes to my office, they're coming into my environment. When I see a patient at home, I'm entering their domain. It gives me a better perspective on who that patient is and allows us to be on a more equal footing. Tina loved it when I visited, and as she got better, she would force-feed me cookies or brownies. I learned to visit with an empty stomach.

Two years later, she was featured in a local newspaper as a living embodiment of her storied retail shop, her warm and dentured smile leaping off the page. Remarkably, Tina went on to live five more years — a testament to the difference that home health care can make for some patients.

I FAIL SCULLY

Scully's tale is a sharp contrast to Debbie and Tina's stories of at-home recovery from hip fractures. Scully was a retired 79-year-old cellist who called me "Bubby." A long-time divorcé, he was diabetic and had slowly progressive Alzheimer's, which I had diagnosed five years earlier. He continued to live alone for the first several years after diagnosis. He had a fondness for General Tso's chicken, which he would order and eat in large quantities, causing his blood sugar level to shoot up.

Both of his children lived far away, so when his diabetes worsened at about age 78, his home care was increased from a few hours to full time, primarily to monitor and control his take-out habits. Things went along in this vein for a while until one fateful morning, when Scully tripped and fell while going for a walk. Taken to the hospital by ambulance, he was found to have a hip fracture, the kind for which no surgery was necessary but bed rest was important.

I spoke to his son and daughter over the phone and asked them to bring Scully home right away.

"Dr. Devi," his son said, "my dad's just fractured his hip. His place is in the hospital, not at home."

In situations like these, where the family and I are at odds, the discussions can turn unpleasant. I gain strength from my sense that I am speaking on behalf of my patient who can no longer advocate for him- or herself. I am also keenly aware that the families are often doing what they think is right, based on what they know to be the medical norm, and that I might be asking them to fly in the face of convention. I outlined my arguments to Scully's children, and they finally, reluctantly agreed to bring him home.

Unfortunately for Scully, his home care agency balked, even though I reassured them that I would supervise the recuperation. They did not want the added risk. From their perspective, Scully was a "high-risk" patient who might fall and reinjure himself. So poor Scully was moved to a rehabilitation facility.

"Bubby," Scully pleaded when I visited him in the facility, "you have got to get me out of this damn place!"

Scully soon became the terror of the floor, refusing to participate in any kind of physical therapy and getting agitated every evening, requiring restraints to tie him down to the bed. Although one of his aides from the agency was with him every day, he still was disoriented and demanded to go home.

He was finally released a month later with nothing to show for it but bedsores — a large one on his lower back and smaller ones on his heels — as well as severe weakness in his legs from the prolonged bed rest and restraints. He never recovered from these injuries and spent nearly all his time in a wheelchair for the last year of his life.

During this year, he became progressively despondent about his condition. His bedsores caused him severe discomfort. His heel sores made walking excruciating, and the less mobile he was, the more pressure there was on these wounds, precluding healing. Scully stopped walking, and was pushed around in a wheelchair by his aides.

"I want to die," he would say to me. "I

don't want to live like this, Bubby."

Antidepressants did not help, and Scully died at 80, after a year of agony. I am convinced that had he been allowed to recuperate with physical therapy at home, he would have been better served. He would have had a vastly better quality of life, not to mention the fact that the costs to society would have been greatly reduced, because his stay, like nearly all inpatient stays of elderly Americans, was covered by Medicare.

REHABILITATING MS. DAISY

Things went somewhat better for my 89-year-old patient Daisy, who had slowly progressive Alzheimer's, with moderate memory impairment and excellent language and life skills. She lived with her husband, who was in his nineties and bed bound with cardiac problems. They shared two full-time aides, with Daisy's aide mainly reminding her to take her medications.

One day, Daisy fell and fractured her hip, needing surgical repair. Her children called to let me know and to ask whether her hip should be pinned under local or general anesthesia. I advocated for local anesthesia, which is associated with a better cognitive outcome than general anesthesia for patients with dementia. This meant that during the surgery Daisy would be sedated and given anesthesia only to the region of the hip.

After the surgery was performed, Daisy's children called to ask what the next step was. I advised them to bring her home right away and to start a regimen of physical therapy there. However, Daisy's surgeon told them to send her to a rehabilitation facility. Torn between two different points of view, the children ultimately decided that Daisy would be better served in a rehab facility.

Once at the facility, Daisy not only refused to walk but refused to get out of bed entirely. She was disoriented and unable to benefit from the rehabilitation. Each time her children called me, the report was worse: Daisy could no longer walk unaided; Daisy could no longer stand without assistance; Daisy refused to sit up in bed. She needed three people to transfer her from bed to wheelchair. She focused on the postoperative pain instead of trying to participate in rehabilitation.

The idea was to get her home when it was "safe," but the longer she stayed there, the less safe it became to send her home. Daisy was finally discharged after two weeks at the facility, during which time she got worse, not better. Once she got home, Daisy slowly recovered over a period of months and eventually was able to walk again, unassisted. But I believe that if Daisy had been sent home immediately after surgery with a visiting physiotherapist, the orienting features and comforting feeling of being in her own home would have motivated her to participate in physical therapy and led to a far speedier recovery.

Going to a rehabilitation facility is often not associated with a better outcome or quicker recovery among patients on the spectrum like Scully or Daisy. The idea of the patient getting "strong" enough to go home often doesn't happen. However, our current health care system is heavily skewed toward facility-based rather than home-based care, making it much easier for families to choose institutional care.

IN THE EVENT OF HOSPITALIZATION

When patients with dementia do end up in the hospital, precautions can be adopted to make the stay beneficial and without deleterious consequences. Most important among these is keeping the length of stay as short as possible, even if it means a little uneasiness at the time of discharge. It's also crucial to stick to taking care of the acute problem that put the patient in the hospital in the first place, rather than trying to fine-tune the patient's overall health.

On countless occasions, a patient who is ready to be discharged is detained a day to perform a test that could just as well be done as an outpatient. Often a family will reason, "A day or two more — what harm can that do?" But every day spent in the hospital, unless absolutely necessary, is a day of additional risk. The patient risks contracting an infection and loses muscle mass from inactivity — which predisposes them to falls, fractures, and rehospitalization. There are also risks associated with procedures and procedure-related complications. Reducing time spent in hospitals is one of the best ways to ensure a "successful" stay — one that has the highest benefit-to-risk ratio.

Despite all the downsides, of course, there are times when the benefits of a hospitalization outweigh the many risks for patients on the Alzheimer's spectrum.

A SUCCESSFUL HOSPITALIZATION

Dr. Packard was a retired 88-year-old surgeon who was referred to me with a diagnosis of Alzheimer's from another neurologist. He came to see me with his

443

wife, Gigi, who was his primary caregiver. A tall, lean man who walked with a distinct limp, Dr. Packard complained about the pain in his right hip every time I saw him.

"Why don't you just take care of my hip and stop worrying about my memory?" he would say.

Gigi told me they had seen two orthopedic surgeons who had agreed that Dr. Packard needed a hip replacement. However, because of his dementia, they thought that surgery was not a good idea. Not only could the surgery and anesthesia worsen his dementia, but because of his cognitive loss, Dr. Packard might not be able to participate in his rehabilitation.

Over the next two years, while Dr. Packard's cognition stabilized on the medication regimen I had started him on, his hip pain progressed to the degree that his complaints about it were almost constant. His face was frequently tightly wound into a distressed grimace. He walked only when absolutely necessary, and when he did, his balance was precarious because his muscles had atrophied from inactivity. I did not give him narcotic analgesics because of the risk of falls and increasing disorientation. We tried many other pain medications, but nothing helped.

Finally, after much discussion and hand-wringing, Dr. Packard, Gigi, and I decided that the time had come for him to have his hip replaced, despite the possible risks. We made this quality-of-life decision after Dr. Packard reached the stage of telling Gigi and me, "I don't want to go on living if it means dealing with this damn pain every day."

I called one of the orthopedic surgeons at the hospital where Dr. Packard had worked before retirement. The surgeon agreed to send Dr. Packard home the morning after his operation, on the condition that he would receive physical therapy and nursing care at home. I thought Dr. Packard's outcome would be improved by reducing his hospital stay to as short a time as possible, with at-home physical therapy in familiar surroundings.

Everything went exactly according to plan. Dr. Packard had his surgery on Monday morning and went home Tuesday morning. A full-time nurse stayed with him for his first two days at home, and a physical therapist visited six times a week to help mobilize Dr. Packard. On his first day home, Gigi called me to let me know that physical therapy had already begun and all was going well. On Friday, she called again to let me know that Dr. Packard was doing much better and was, in fact, far less irritable because he was no longer in pain. Most surprising of all, Gigi claimed that his memory loss had improved. I found this hard to believe.

Sure enough, when I saw Dr. Packard three weeks after his hip surgery, he walked into my office with a wide smile, and his memory was in fact better. Although he still had Alzheimer's, his memory had improved overall from the moderate level to the mild level. I learned two things that day: One was to never underestimate a patient's complaint of pain. The second was that pain can have a significant effect on cognitive ability. These facts seem so obvious now, almost in the "Duh!" category of realizations, but at the time, it was far from clear. We had attributed a lot of Dr. Packard's confusion to his dementia, when, in fact, it was from his severe, daily pain.

Amelia, a 90-year-old patient who had slowly progressive Alzheimer's, also had a hip fracture that was treated successfully in a hospital.

Even after the onset of dementia, Amelia could speak four different languages fluently — Hungarian, French, German, and English — and she managed all of her daily self-care activities. Amelia's daughter, a pediatrician, initially had brought her mother to see me about her dementia. However, I quickly became concerned because Amelia was preoccupied with her hip pain. Having learned my lesson from Dr. Packard nearly a decade before, I had her assessed orthopedically. The surgeon concluded that Amelia needed a hip replacement.

Before the surgery, we made it very clear that she was to receive only local anesthesia and would need to go home soon afterward. However, Amelia's surgeon thought the complexity of the surgery required general anesthesia and that she would need a few days of hospitalization.

Based on our discussions, Amelia's daughter got her a private room and filled it with music that her mother liked. In addition, she and her sister took turns staying with Amelia around the clock, sleeping there, talking to her throughout the day, and keeping her oriented. They also made sure that physical therapy started right away. Amelia was able to transition home after three days. For the first week, Amelia worked with a physical therapist who made home visits. She was then able to participate in a physical therapy program at a nearby facility. Her walking has been fine ever since. In fact, because of the severity of her memory impairment, Amelia has no recollection of the surgery even taking place.

I believe both Dr. Packard and Amelia's stories had positive outcomes because we were able to take them both home quickly.

HOME IS ALMOST ALWAYS THE BETTER OPTION

Although some patients and families may find such scenarios of treating patients at home implausible or unfeasible, home care is a real option. Home care nursing and home physical therapy are covered by insurance and cost taxpayers far fewer Medicare dollars than recuperation in an inpatient rehabilitation facility. More important, they are associated with a better outcome for the patient. It is a win-win situation, and I only wish such scenarios were more common.

My aim with these stories is not to denigrate hospitals. Obviously, there are patients with dementia who are alive today because of appropriate hospitalization and the expert care rendered there. Instead, I am advocating for carefully thinking through whether a hospital is the best place for a particular patient with dementia. This runs counter to our instinctive sense that hospitals are the best places to get to health from illness. However, as my experiences with my patients have illustrated, it is my firm belief that for patients with dementia, management at home is a preferable option, and makes for better medical care.

The idea of having a patient stay home when they have an emergency instead of opting to call 911 can be terrifying for a family. Sometimes there is conflict between family members over what the best course of action is. To avoid these conflicts, it's helpful to discuss the patient's wishes for emergency situations when they are well. What would they prefer? Would they rather be home if they had a treatable medical illness, even if the hospital could provide superior care? Just because a patient is on the Alzheimer's spectrum does not mean they cannot comprehend and give logical answers to such questions. I have had countless discussions like this over the years with patients, even those with severe memory loss. As long as their language abilities are preserved, patients are able to clearly let me know what they want. In families with several involved members, it is important that they're all on board with the decision. All of this needs to be documented with a living will and appropriate designation of health care proxies, as we will read in Chapter 15.

A discussion with the patient's primary physician or internist is also crucial. Is he or she amenable to the plan? Or do they favor a hospital-based approach? Some physicians may believe in the efficacy of home care but opt for hospitals, as we are all increasingly pressed for time. Caring for a patient with dementia at home is time intensive for physicians and poorly reimbursed by insurance companies and Medicare.

Ultimately, both families and physicians want to do what is in the best interests of the patient. It's best to plan ahead and prepare for medical emergencies so obstacles can be anticipated and addressed in advance, and so that regrettable decisions are not made in moments of haste.

CHAPTER 14
WHETHER YOU LIKE IT OR NOT, HERE'S WHAT I WANT.
MAINTAINING INDIVIDUALITY IN THE FACE OF ALZHEIMER'S

Often, when people get diagnosed with Alzheimer's, all their eccentricities — and all of us are eccentric in one way or another — become pathologized. Their quirks and preferences are now deemed by caregivers to be part and parcel of the Alzheimer's diagnosis and therefore targets for elimination.

I find this attitude very difficult to accept. In a society that's increasingly moving toward medical and personal conformity and homogeneity, we don't allow patients the individual quirks that make them the men and women they are. People with Alzheimer's are as entitled to their unorthodox choices as people without Alzheimer's. Some of us maintain tidy homes, others are messy. Some of us are savers, others spend-thrifts. Some of us coddle our dogs, and others dislike pets. We carry our preferences into old age and dementia. When our friends, family, and coworkers try to impose their preferences on us — and we don't have a diagnosis of Alzheimer's — we say "Pshaw" and move on. Our friends and family shake their heads in frustration but rarely try to override our foibles. Unfortunately, when patients with Alzheimer's have nonconformist tendencies, family and caregivers rationalize the sweeping away of a patient's preferences by attributing such unpalatable behaviors to dementia.

It's important to remember what the patient was like before the onset of dementia. There are Alzheimer's patients who used to be meticulous but now are sloppy, and those who never gave a damn about being well ordered. The key word here is *before*. Was this quirk evident prior to their diagnosis? Answering this question helps distinguish individual preference from changes caused by Alzheimer's disease, although it's not a foolproof guide by any means, because of a critical caveat: Our tastes change.

We all evolve over time, and our tastes and our preferences follow suit. If you had told me twenty years ago that one day I would weep over the beauty of a mezzo-soprano singing an aria, I would have laughed you out of the room. Of course, this is a relatively innocuous change in preferences. But what happens when a previously devoted husband becomes a lothario in his sixties after a divorce? If the same man later develops a dementia in his eighties, his gallivanting cannot then be ascribed to his dementia.

A PRINCE OR A PUP?

Thomas, 90, was a patient whose eccentricities were difficult to classify. He had slowly progressive Alzheimer's, with mild to moderate memory loss, excellent language skills, and mild living skills impairment. I had met and diagnosed Thomas more than a decade previously, when he was 79, and in the intervening years, I got to know his habits well.

I discovered, for example, from a physical therapist I sent to his apartment, that Thomas's home was a very messy place, covered in piles of papers and with dog feces in evidence. It was unclear to me if his poor housekeeping was the result of his Alzheimer's or a preexisting tendency. I discussed it with Thomas, and he assured me that he had a housekeeper who came to clean three days a week and that he had always been "messy with my papers."

At six feet five inches tall, Thomas had a large gut that remained valiantly and stubbornly slung low over his belt, jauntily resistant to my decade-long efforts to put him on a diet. Thomas continued his nightly snack of a pint of Ben & Jerry's Cherry Garcia ice cream. A longtime classics professor at a small liberal arts college, he had lived alone for almost all of his life, and strongly resisted conforming to conventional notions of what was acceptable and what was not. He made no apologies for his preferences.

"Ask me again when I'm awake," Thomas often said when I started my examination by inquiring into his health. "This is too early for me."

"But Thomas," I protested, "it's two o'clock in the afternoon!"

I learned over time that Thomas went to bed around 3:00 a.m., an hour or two after his de rigueur pint of Cherry Garcia, and awoke at about one in the afternoon. I learned to accommodate his routine, scheduling his visits for the late afternoon.

Thomas lived with a little Chihuahua named Prince. Now, I love dogs — in my lifetime, I have been lucky enough to care for more than two dozen, and I appreciate varied canine personalities. But Prince was a piece of work by anyone's standards.

Thomas adopted Prince from a rescue

organization, despite the fact that the dog was anxious and prone to nipping at everything in sight — the reason he had been given up by his previous owner. This foible of Prince's did not faze Thomas one bit. The one person Prince never tried to harm was Thomas, whom he adored with all the fierce loyalty of a rescued dog.

Prince was Thomas's main companion and stayed next to him at all times. Only Thomas could get along with this feisty, snappy little dog, and they developed a particularly strong bond. Thomas would come to my office and spend much of his time talking about Prince. He told me he had given the Chihuahua that name because Prince had a noble bearing and, much like royalty, Prince did not "deign to consort with the proletariat."

"I find him refreshingly old-fashioned," Thomas observed with contentment. "None of this modern 'reaching out.' "

Sadly, after some time, Prince suffered an accident that broke his spine. Now, not only was Prince nippy, but he was also confined to a little contraption for his hind legs so he could get around. As Thomas's dementia progressed, he was unable to take very good care of Prince, who needed to be catheterized every so often to allow his urine to drain. Thomas said that he never forgot to do that, but I was unsure and worried that the little dog might not be getting the care he needed. At a certain point, I decided to involve a home care agency to help Thomas and to help Thomas help Prince.

The agency staff was as appalled by Thomas's living situation as the visiting physical therapist had been previously, complaining about the dog poop and stacks of paper. Both his housekeeper of twenty-five years and I tried to assure them that this was Thomas's way, that although the height of the piles of paper may have worsened with his dementia, they had been high to begin with. This was his home, and it was how Thomas had always liked it.

"We need someone to go in there and clean up the mess," the agency representative said, despite my assurances. "This can't be healthy."

"It's never reached the point of being a health hazard," I said. "His housekeeper is there a few days a week and cleans everything up. He doesn't like his stacks of papers moved."

The agency staff was not persuaded by my arguments and thought that this was no way for a civilized human to live. They cleaned Thomas's apartment and put away his ubiquitous piles of paper. This disoriented him — he believed he had been moved to a different apartment, because his home, in its newly immaculate state, was unrecognizable to him. Not only that, but after all this perturbation, he also inexplicably failed to recognize Prince as his own dog.

Thomas told me, "I have a new dog."

"Oh?" I said. "What's his name?"

"Pup," he told me.

"How old is Pup?" I asked.

"Pup's only two years old."

I asked what had happened to Prince.

Thomas said, "I'm not sure, but I think they replaced Prince with Pup."

"How do you know? What's going on with Pup?"

He said that Pup had the same contraption for his back legs that Prince had had.

I asked, "Well, how do you know that Pup isn't Prince?"

Thomas replied, "I know my Prince. My Prince was aristocratic, he was nobility. Pup is just a pup."

About a month after my ill-fated call to the home care agency, their staff took Prince to the pound because of his nippy personality. Given Prince's diminutive size and paralysis, he had always been an annoyance rather than a true threat. Even so, the agency staff did not take kindly to Prince and had removed him.

Thomas may have had memory loss, but this was no match for his love for his dog. When told that the little dog had gotten "lost," Pup suddenly morphed back into Prince in Thomas's mind. Despite his memory loss, Thomas recalled that Prince had a microchip and made the required calls, locating his Prince in the shelter and rescuing him yet again.

Thomas's family, who lived far away, grew tired of the near daily complaints about Prince from the home care agency staff. They had the dog removed and placed outside the shelter system. The family believed they were doing the right thing, and with regard to Prince's welfare, perhaps they were. It had been a difficult life for Prince. However, I didn't think it was the right thing for Thomas. After Prince was removed, Thomas had a longer, sadder face than I had ever seen in my many years of knowing him.

"I don't know what happened to my Prince," he told me. "My mind must be so far gone that I let him wander away from me. The last thing I remember, I was walking Prince, and the next thing I know, there's no Prince in the apartment. I must have lost him. I've called all the shelters and no one has him."

He was tortured by this. "I don't know what I'm going to do without him," he said sadly. "He was my life; he was my companion."

I wondered aloud whether someone had taken Prince because he was so cute. Thomas laughed. "Dr. Devi," he said, "you and I both know that Prince was nobody's darling but mine. Nobody's going to want him. I hope he's somewhere safe."

Thomas died a year after all this, after a colonoscopy — which I had opposed — and a five-day hospital stay, preparing for and recovering from the procedure. He left the hospital with trouble walking and within weeks after his colonoscopy, he was spending nearly all his waking hours in a wheelchair. He then had several more hospitalizations for an infection, although I argued that he should be treated at home for them. My recommendations were met with incredulity by his family, who eventually replaced me with a physician who was, in their opinion, more sane. I found out about Thomas's death from the psychiatrist who had initially referred him to me.

To be fair, Thomas's other two physicians,

his psychiatrist and his internist, were in complete agreement with the home care agency's plan of action; it seemed sensible and healthy to them. I was the odd person out. But I believe that, had Thomas not had Alzheimer's, we all might have tolerated his living situation. Because Thomas had the diagnosis, it gave both family and health care workers the power to impose an external set of values.

I remember in one of my last conversations with him, Thomas told me, "I cannot comprehend the idea of my nonexistence." Although he is no longer with us, his story continues to linger in my mind. Like all of us, patients with Alzheimer's need a sense of purpose in life, and I believe Thomas's was Prince. Losing his dog was a difficult blow from which to recover and was compounded by numerous hospitalizations — five in the last year of his life.

The difficulty in Thomas's situation was differentiating behaviors attributable to Alzheimer's from those that were inherent to Thomas. Were the piles of stacked papers a long-standing Thomas habit, or were there unread pieces of mail and unpaid bills in them, as can happen with patients with dementia? Was the dog feces in the house the result of Thomas's relaxed attitude toward cleanliness or a symptom of his Alzheimer's? In both instances, based on historical information, the answer seemed to be Thomas rather than his dementia.

Of course, even if Thomas had always kept stacks of paper around his apartment, having unpaid bills in the stacks would have needed sorting out. In this case, I'd have advocated for handling the situation with discreet sensitivity and tact, not yielding to the temptation of "let's-convert-Thomas-into-a-neatnik." My approach to taking care of patients with Alzheimer's disease is not the norm in the medical community. But if I developed Alzheimer's, I'd want my idiosyncrasies to be accepted.

A Special Request

Estelle had rapidly progressive Alzheimer's with mild memory loss and significant language difficulties. At 91, she had spent the entirety of her life in a small, affluent New Jersey town, married to her high school sweetheart for sixty-five years until his death. She had raised two daughters, who had brought her to me shortly after I started my practice. I had been seeing her for a few months when, one afternoon, she felt the need to confess something to me.

"I have had a good life . . . but I still want

one thing," she tried to explain. "I've never had it. I've never had this thing."

Estelle was tinier than she had been as a young woman, thanks to osteoporosis corroding her spine. Even so, she sat firmly in her chair, her eyes carefully lined in black eyeliner, her eyebrows similarly well drawn, determinedly trying to explain herself. Estelle's daughters had originally brought her to see me because Estelle was having trouble finding words. As her dementia progressed, she struggled more and more to form complete sentences. Nonetheless, Estelle was insistent on being heard, and I tried hard to understand what she was saying that afternoon.

"That thing," Estelle said. "You can get someone for it. Can't you get me someone for it? There are people who can help you get it."

"I'm not sure what you're talking about. What do you mean?" I kept asking.

"You know," she tried again, looking directly at me. "When you're in bed . . ."

Bed? I sensed she was trying to tell me about something related to sex, not sleep, but I had no inkling what it was. I also had to work through my own discomfort. How could I possibly discuss sex with someone as old as my great-grandmother?

But as Estelle tried to get the words out, I realized that if she could make this courageous leap, I should be able to hang on to her hem and take the leap with her. It took a while to figure it out, but it finally dawned on me that Estelle was talking about climaxing.

"An orgasm?" I asked, delighted to have figured out the riddle and a little shocked at the same time.

"Yes!" she said. "Yes, that's it! An orgasm! Can't you get me somebody for it? For money? A man? A prostitute?"

As we spoke, it became clear to me that Estelle had never had an orgasm. It was something she was curious about and wanted to experience. She hadn't told anyone this before, perhaps because she thought she was going to be judged. I'm glad she somehow knew that I wouldn't respond that way. I didn't find her request off-putting or repugnant — I found it surprising, but poignant nonetheless, and I was grateful that she trusted me enough to open up about such a private topic. Doctors, like priests and teachers, are able to be part of such intensely intimate moments if they are receptive to it.

"Do your daughters know about this?" I asked, already sure that they did not.

"No, no!" Estelle said, and burst into laughter.

"Do you want me to tell them, to see if we can make it happen?"

Estelle nodded eagerly.

I invited her daughters into my office, hopeful that we could make Estelle's dream a reality. In the exuberance of the discovery, I didn't anticipate her daughters' response, but perhaps Estelle did. Maybe this was the reason for her suddenly somber attitude: She was sitting beside me with a serious expression on her face, but I failed to recognize the change in her mood.

"I asked your mom's permission to be able to tell you this, and she gave me her blessing," I said to her two daughters. "I think she wants us to help her achieve a certain goal . . ."

We told them — two women in their sixties, grandmothers themselves — about their mother's wishes. One daughter was a social worker, fighting valiantly with aging, visibly nipped, tucked, and dyed, and the other daughter was a dancer who was letting nature take root, graying and spreading comfortably.

"How dare you?" the social worker yelled into the silence that followed my announcement, wiping a happy grin off my face.

"That is so *in . . . inappropriate.* How could you even discuss such a thing with my mother? It's my mom you're talking about here. You're her neurologist, not her pimp. I thought you were doing a neurologic examination in there, not talking nonsense. I cannot believe you brought this up! Simply disgusting!"

I landed back on earth with a thud and found that Estelle was already there, waiting for me. Estelle said nothing; she just looked quietly at the floor.

The dancer daughter tried to intervene. "If Mom feels like this . . ." she began.

Her sister was having none of it. "Oh, for heaven's sake, Sue, stop it!" she said. "We came here to have Mom treated for her memory by a doctor, not to get her laid by a prostitute!"

That was that, end of discussion. There was nothing more I could do. After all, as a neurologist, it was not my role to facilitate the procurement of orgasms. All these years later, I still recall the gentle touch of Estelle's hand on my arm at that moment, imperceptible to the others, a small thank-you that left the spirit in me even as we both lost that battle and Estelle lost her war.

THE JUDGE AND THE
NOBEL LAUREATE

I have kept Estelle's story a secret in my professional life until now. It seemed so sordid in immediate retrospect, and yet, looking back now, it seems more tragic than anything else. But vindication of my approach arrived nearly two decades later in the unlikely habitus of a tall and distinguished professor, who also happened to have won a Nobel Prize in medicine.

How gratifying to discover that Dr. Nobel Laureate agreed with my stance on allowing patients with Alzheimer's to do whatever they needed to live out their last years happily. In fact, he was actively engaged in helping his dear friend Judge Gavin do just that. The judge, 85 and long retired, had developed memory loss over six years, and I diagnosed him with slowly progressive Alzheimer's with moderate memory loss and mild living skills and language loss.

Judge Gavin was a brilliant man who had been married many times, thanks to his wandering eye and fondness for curves. He and his current wife lived in a gigantic, turn-of-the-last-century mansion in the old-money section of Greenwich, Connecticut, surrounded by pavilions and pools and acres and acres of landscaped wilderness.

As his wife discovered her husband's progressing dementia, she began to try to have his finances reapportioned in her favor. Judge Gavin, though, was still savvy and refused to have any of it. He may have had dementia, but he wanted to retain control of his money, especially since he had not much trusted Wife Number Six to begin with.

Knowing that his memory was deteriorating, Judge Gavin designated Dr. Nobel Laureate, his longtime friend and confidant, as his health care proxy, and gave another friend his financial power of attorney.

Eventually, the situation with Wife Number Six came to a head and became quite unpleasant for the judge. There were constant fights, raised voices, and slammed doors; his wife even displayed some physical aggression toward Judge Gavin — not serious, but enough to be concerning.

The funny thing is that when the judge mentioned these troubles, he would add with a smile, "Yes, she's after my money and thinks of no one but herself. But boy! That body!" He would say this with a wink of his lively eyes as he rubbed his hands together.

It was clear that he still enjoyed having her in his life. She gave him purpose — in a negative way, perhaps, but purpose never-theless.

One day, I got a call from Dr. Nobel Laureate.

"Everything has been arranged," he informed me. "There is going to be a court-mandated separation between the judge and his missus, and she's going to move out. The judge wanted her out and the courts agreed with him. I think things will be much better at home — the judge will finally have some peace."

My heart sank when I heard this news. I was sure that the primary reason Judge Gavin was still so engaged with life was that he had his metaphorical boxing gloves at the ready. The ongoing fights with his nubile and conniving young wife kept him going. I feared that taking that away from him would destroy his zest for living.

I began to allude to my concern as delicately as possible during my conversation with Judge Gavin's eminent trustee. I did so with a great deal of trepidation. It's hard enough to be ridiculed by one's colleagues for one's beliefs, but to be laughed at by a Nobel Laureate would be particularly bruising to the ego.

But Dr. Laureate immediately understood my oblique references and got straight to the point. "I've thought about that," he said. "But don't worry, *I'm procuring him a courtesan.*"

At first I couldn't believe my ears. When I was sure I had heard right, I asked him how one would go about doing such a thing.

"There are places," Dr. Laureate replied, "like Palm Beach, for example. I think we've located just the right person to keep the old boy on his toes."

"I'm so happy that you think like this," I said, delighted and laughing with relief. "I've felt alone in my outlook, so it's nice to have an imprimatur from someone as celebrated as yourself."

Dr. Laureate turned out to be the best person to help Judge Gavin. He did not see this time as an opportunity to redeem the wayward ways of his friend, as so many concerned family members might have been wont to do in similar circumstances. Instead, he carried out the essence of his responsibility, what he had been entrusted and charged with — Dr. Laureate helped maintain his ward's quality of life in the way that the judge himself would've chosen. *No wonder he won a Nobel Prize,* I thought to myself. *The man is a genius!*

How Purple Is Too Purple?

Not all patients are as fortunate as Judge Gavin. Constance was 91 when I saw her for the first time. I diagnosed her with slowly progressive Alzheimer's, with mild-moderate memory loss and good language and life skills. She was a small, delicate woman, around five feet two inches. She reminded me of a hummingbird — full of frenetic energy, hands fluttering constantly and often straying to her hair, which was a brilliant shade of blue. In the six years that I knew her, her hair became progressively bluer, eventually turning an exuberant purplish shade not readily found in nature. The changing shades were the result of her love for her 72-year-old hairdresser, Eddie.

Constance visited her hair salon as many as three times a week, and each time, she tipped her love a large amount. I came to realize that Eddie was a great source of joy for Constance — she was excited and upbeat throughout the week because of her visits with him.

One day I got a call from her daughter, Amy. "Mother is spending too much money at the hair salon!" she declared. "I really don't want her going to see her stylist anymore. She is infatuated and keeps saying that she wants to marry him."

"Well, do you really think that's going to happen?" I asked.

Constance's daughter didn't find my question amusing.

"Mother is a very wealthy woman," she told me sternly. "And this man knows it. He's taking advantage of her."

"Amy," I replied, "your mother needs some pleasure in her life, which is what Eddie provides. She can certainly afford her salon visits. Does the relatively small amount she spends there really matter in the grand scheme of things, when it gives her such joy?"

Our conversation went nowhere, and eventually, Amy hung up on me. By that time, I had learned a lot about Constance, and she had become one of my favorite patients. I knew that when she was a young mother, Constance doted on her two children and tended toward lavish gestures. She once told me, "I decided I had to give my son Jack a present he would remember for his eighteenth birthday. So I told my Harry" — her husband, who had since died — "that I wanted to get Jack something really special. Harry thought I was crazy, but I got Jack a convertible that was delivered to the street outside our apartment building."

When her son woke up, Constance excitedly told Jack to look out his window. There, right on the avenue, he saw a shiny red sports car tied up with a big yellow ribbon. He was so happy, it didn't even matter to him that he didn't yet know how to drive. "He got his license in two months," Constance said, smiling.

Constance was generous like that with both of her children. But she revealed that as the years went by, her children had become very involved in her finances. They didn't approve of the way she spent her money.

"My Harry was not like that," Constance told me. "He used to say, 'Spend well and live well, just don't spend beyond your means.' I don't understand my children. I don't understand why they turned out like this. I don't even think they love me very much," she added sadly.

As time went on, Constance became aware that her children, who were both quite well off in their own right, were suspicious of her beloved hairdresser.

"They think Eddie's after my money," she told me in a whisper. "Of course, he's after a little bit of my money. Who isn't? And who cares? He's been my hairdresser for more than twenty years, and I know I really mean something to him. If he wanted money from me, he could've taken advantage of me long ago. He's never done that because he's a wonderful man. I wouldn't be in love with him if he wasn't."

Constance would look at me with her bright eyes, under a fringe of purple hair, and it was impossible not to love her pixie spirit. I remember that my dog Max once nipped at Constance's daughter. I was horrified and scolded Max, now long departed, who had never done such a thing before or since. I remember Constance telling me, "Leave him alone. Max clearly is a good judge of character."

Meanwhile, unbeknownst to both Constance and myself, her children had put her lovely five-bedroom apartment on Park Avenue, where she had lived for more than seventy years, up for sale. She came to my office in tears once she found out.

"They're sending me away," she said, weeping. "I'm going to a nursing home. I don't know how they did it. I called my lawyer and he says I signed papers for this. I don't remember doing it. My own children are forcing me out of my home."

I was dismayed. Worse still, I never saw or heard from Constance again. I understood, based on the medical records requested, that she had been moved to a nursing home in Connecticut.

Constance's wishes were simple: All she wanted was to stay in her own home and keep getting her hair done a few times a week. The relationship with Eddie was important for Constance, for her sense of well-being. Parenthetically, in going to her hairdresser as often as she did, Constance was also meeting her human need for being touched by another human being whom she cared about, and who she believed cared about her. The impersonal, "task-oriented" touch of a hairdresser had evolved for Constance, over the length of their relationship, into the caring, nurturing touch of her Eddie. Older patients can sometimes go for weeks, months, or even years without the feel of another person's skin on theirs, aside from impersonal touches. This is the saddest kind of deprivation. Unfortunately, her children did not understand it.

When I witness stories like these, I think about how important it is to select the right people to make decisions on one's behalf. Close relatives like spouses and children seem the obvious choices, but they may not always be the right ones.

Although Constance's children seemed uncaring to me, sometimes even very caring children and caregivers can make mistakes, as Ella's daughter nearly did.

A Younger Man

"Ninety-eight is too much. Ninety-eight is *too much,*" said my patient Ella for what seemed to me the ninety-eighth time. She said this every time she came to see me, referring of course to her age. A former professor of music, she had slowly progressive Alzheimer's with moderate to severe memory loss. She was aware that she had authored numerous books on music and culture, but she could not remember the names of any of them or what they were about, although some of them were still in print forty years later.

"If you can give me something to take so that I can go to sleep and not wake up anymore, that would be perfect. I know you can't, but I wish you would," she said to me at least twice each time I saw her. "I've had my turn. I've had a wonderful life. I have been *admired,* and that can never be underestimated. I have a daughter whom I adore and who adores me. I have a man in my life. That's pretty good, don't you think, at ninety-eight? To have a loving daughter and a loving man?" Ella chuckled. "Not bad! I'm not complaining. But ninety-eight is too much."

475

Ella had an enviable quality of life. Her gentleman friend, also a former professor, lived a block away from her in Greenwich Village. He was, Ella ecstatically exclaimed, "Elegant! Aristocratic! Refined!" And at 92, he was "a younger man"! Each week, they spent four days together in her residence and three days apart in their respective homes. This arrangement had worked well for them for nearly sixteen years, but as Ella's dementia progressed, her daughter, Lynn, became upset with the situation.

"He's abusive to my mother," she told me. "He yells and screams. I want him out of her life."

"Have they always had such a contentious relationship?" I asked.

"Yes," Lynn admitted. "I don't understand how she has stayed with him. I want to stop him from ever being with her again. It breaks my heart the way he carries on."

I asked Ella about this when I next saw her. "No, no," she said. "I would never abide a man who was abusive to me. I love myself too much. We have very heated arguments, that is true. That is our way of discussing things — the opera, movies, you name it."

I called Lynn. "This man adds value to your mother's life and gives her a sense of well-being," I told her. "Don't take that

476

away from her."

Lynn reluctantly agreed, despite her uneasiness with the situation. She acknowledged that there had never been any hint of physical abuse and agreed to stay out of this aspect of her mother's life. I was obviously not able to grant Ella her wish of a death potion, and she grudgingly lives on, heading toward 100. But I am happy to have been able to help her keep her textured, possibly tortured relationship alive, and with it, her quality of life.

Respecting Preferences in Dementia

What we each want out of life as we get older is as unpredictable and varied as the people in this world. Regardless of whether we have Alzheimer's, we all make inexplicable choices related to our likes and dislikes. Some patients' choices may result from the effects of the illness, but others may be a reflection of who they intrinsically are as a person. It can sometimes be difficult to distinguish between the two, and at such times, it is helpful to know more about a patient's past life and preferences, before they developed dementia.

To get a sense of the person behind an illness, it's important to try to equalize the power dynamic inherent in a doctor-patient relationship. This is particularly true when dealing with Alzheimer's patients, who may be more diffident as the result of their compromised cognition, and therefore even more vulnerable to perceived power shifts. When the relationship feels more equitable, it creates a safe space where the patient can speak openly not only about treatment preferences, but also about themselves. This allows the physician an additional window into the mind of the patient and more opportunities to be helpful. I try my best to prevent patients from feeling intimidated. Particularly in situations where a patient's wishes are unorthodox, it is imperative that the patient and the physician are on that most equal footing of two human beings communicating with each other.

On the other side, it can be hard on caregivers and families to find the resources within themselves to tolerate behavior vastly different from theirs, particularly when such behavior is highly idiosyncratic. But supporting the wishes of Alzheimer's patients and refraining from adopting a reformist attitude — the kind of attitude that led to Thomas losing his Princely Pup — is essential for helping them live with dignity. Even on the occasions when we cannot fulfill the wishes of the patients, as with Estelle, it's important to maintain sensitivity.

Chapter 15
I Would Rather Die at Home. Living and Dying with Dignity — in the Comfort of Home

I used to wonder what makes for a good physician. Does it mean being a great diagnostician? Does it mean caring about the patient? Does it mean being able to choose the right treatment? I have come to the conclusion that these abilities are important for all physicians, but depending on the specialty, other variables need to be considered. A pediatrician who was caring and smart but had a tough time dealing with the inherent messiness of children would have a difficult time of it, for example. In specialties dealing with chronic illness, I believe a good physician, in addition to supporting patients in their efforts at better health, also will help them die with as little pain and as much dignity as possible. In other words, a good physician will help his or her patients die a "good" death.

For me, a good death means dying where we want, surrounded by those we want, and sometimes, if we are lucky, when and how we want. Eighty percent of Americans — based on polls and palliative care data — want to die at home, but 80 percent of us will, in fact, die in hospitals and nursing homes. This is particularly true for dementia patients. In fact, the number of those placed in hospitals or intensive care units in the last three months of life is on the rise.

Guiding patients on the Alzheimer's spectrum to a "good" death, when that time comes, involves a great deal of pragmatic planning. Sometimes it involves preventing them from getting to the hospital in the first place, by treating illness at home. It also involves having ongoing discussions with the patient and the family about their wishes regarding hospitalization and nursing home placement, and writing out advanced directives or living wills so that the wishes are clearly delineated. Being deliberate in this fashion prevents panic and chaos when crucial decisions need to be made quickly. For example, should a family member call 911 when a 92-year-old relative on the spectrum with severe memory and life skill loss has fallen and cannot get up? Such what-if scenarios are best discussed ahead of time. My thinking has been guided by

481

certain formative experiences I had early in my career.

A TOUGH STICK

I'll never forget my sad first lesson in elder care in the intensive care unit. Still in medical school, I was doing a general surgery rotation and had to draw arterial blood from a tiny 94-year-old woman who had been admitted for lung cancer. For a week, she had been unresponsive in the ICU, with a tube in her throat connected to a respirator. She had multiple intravenous lines in her arms and neck.

I remember my senior resident telling me, "I need you to get ABGs [arterial blood gases] from this patient." He added, "She's a tough stick," meaning difficult to get blood from, "and I don't care what you have to do, just get them."

The patient, frail as she was, had had both arms poked so many times in the last ten days, and her wrists were swollen and bruised to such a degree, that I couldn't feel her pulse anywhere. She had been having these ABGs done several times a day so that the settings on her respirator could be changed. The difficulty finding her arteries was compounded by my inexperience. I must have stuck her with a needle eight times to get that blood gas for my resident. I felt sick thinking how much I must have hurt her, and I prayed that, unconscious as she was, she didn't feel it. Her ABGs came back fine, and I remember feeling immensely relieved, because if they hadn't, I would have had to stick her again later that night. But it was all futile anyway. She died the next day.

As a result of this vivid experience, as I climbed up the medical ladder, becoming an intern, resident, and then chief resident, I was careful not to order such tests in the elderly unless absolutely necessary.

THE RIGHT HUMAN DECISION

Early in my medical training, when I was living and working in Brooklyn, I befriended my elderly next door neighbor, Annie. She taught me another lesson that has guided me throughout my professional life.

Annie was a petite, 92-year-old firecracker of a woman with a spine curved over like a question mark from osteoporosis. Wearing a blue housecoat, she liked to station herself at the parlor floor window of her brownstone — the same brownstone she was born in — and watch the goings-on of our block from morning until evening. She had no surviving family other than a niece who lived in Boston.

Every morning and evening on my way to and from work, I'd pass her window and wave. My husband and I were juggling work and caring for our young daughter, but when I had free time, I'd sometimes pay Annie a visit. She had no visitors other than the neighborhood priest, and very occasionally her niece, so Annie very much enjoyed company. I'd take my daughter with me and we'd sit in Annie's basement kitchen, where she'd regale us with stories of her childhood and her six brothers, who all became police officers. She enjoyed gossiping about her neighbors, especially about the priest across the street and how she would sometimes see women going into his home.

"What business does he have with these women?" Annie would whisper, as if my daughter could understand the implication.

Sometimes, she would tell me about the people down the street. "I saw him kick his dog," she would say about another neighbor. "He's a mean man, if you ask me. . . ."

Because her niece was farther away, I became Annie's de facto caregiver. Knowing I was a resident doctor, she decided to make me her medical sounding board, although I was never directly involved in her care. She would bring out all of her medications during my visits and line them up on the kitchen table, aghast.

"Look at what those morons gave me today!" she would complain. "They expect me to take this nonsense?"

Then she would sweep the pill bottles off the Formica kitchen table in one grand motion.

"Annie!" I'd protest. "These drugs are important for keeping you healthy." I scrambled to the floor to pick up the pill containers.

With a thumb pointed to her chest, Annie would shake her head and say, "The only reason I have lived this long is that I stayed away from your kind of people. No doctors for me, thank you very much. None of these drugs either. They only make me feel bad."

I enjoyed visiting Annie, not only because I knew she looked forward to our time together, but also because I loved her sense of humor, the sparkle in her eyes, and her zest. I made a habit of bringing along her favorite treat: sugared jelly doughnuts. I got a kick out of watching her and my small daughter sitting side by side, each loudly and gleefully sucking the jelly out of them.

As time went on, I could see that Annie was developing progressive heart failure. Her ankles were swollen and she was increasingly short of breath, even on the brief walk from the kitchen to the front door to let us in. She started sleeping on the couch in the dining room so she wouldn't have to climb the stairs to her parlor floor bedroom. She remained as stubborn as a goat, though. Nothing I ever said could persuade her to take her medications.

After one visit, I phoned her niece, Diana, to let her know that her aunt's health was deteriorating.

"She's not doing well, Diana," I said.

"Yes, I know!" she replied. "She refuses to listen to me, her doctors, or anyone else. This has always been her way — as stubborn as the day is long. What can I do?"

The next time I stopped by, I could barely hear Annie's weak voice from her kitchen when I knocked on the door. I let myself in, as Annie had left the door unlocked. I found her hunched over her kitchen table, barely able to breathe. She was wheezing badly, and I saw that she was gravely ill.

She looked at me from where she still slumped on the yellow Formica table. "I want to die here," she managed to say. "Don't you call anyone! I want to die right here, in my home."

I didn't know what to do. I was a mere resident, a few years out of school, and I didn't have the experience and the knowledge I do now. I was aware that Annie needed help, but I also knew, even back then, that the help wasn't going to keep her alive. She was 92, had serious medical issues, and was not given to complying with treatment. Even if she was successfully treated and discharged from a hospital, her prognosis was grim. But it was not my place to make that decision.

I called Diana from the house. "Your aunt is really ill," I said. "I don't think she's going to make it through the night. She wants to stay here at home. What would you like me to do?"

"Call 911," Diana said. "I'll be there as soon as possible."

Annie was watching me from the corners of her eyes. "Don't do it," she whispered. "I want to die here. I don't want to go to a hospital. Please," she pleaded. "*You* can take care of me!"

"Annie, I'm sorry," I told her. My heart was breaking. "I'm a neurologist in training. I don't know how to take care of you."

I did as Diana asked and called 911. The ambulance sirens split the calm evening air, the flashing lights visible through Annie's kitchen window. The last time I saw her, she was being lifted on a stretcher into the back of the ambulance, her blue housecoat flapping in the wind. Just before they closed the doors to drive her away, Annie sat bolt upright in the ambulance, screaming to me, "They're gonna kill me! They're gonna kill me! Don't let them take me away! Don't you let them take me away!"

Annie died in the hospital about a week after that, as she predicted, never returning home. I tried very hard not to imagine what her last week was like, how often she was poked with needles. I imagined her small hands swollen. I imagined her sedated because of her "combative" behavior.

It wasn't hard to picture. I saw people like Annie at my hospital every day, but this was *my* Annie, and *I* had done this to her. If I hadn't visited her that evening, maybe she would have died at home without all the tragedy of her last days in the hospital. I had made the right medical decision, but had I made the right human decision?

In time, I came to believe that the right medical decision had to be the right human decision. I didn't realize how fervently committed I was to this principle until I got a call seven years later. I was, by then, a full-fledged neurologist with my own thriving practice.

The phone rang one Tuesday afternoon. It was Luke, the husband of one of my favorite patients, Polly. He told me she was throwing up blood.

Polly was 84 and had dementia because of both Alzheimer's and strokes, with mild-moderate memory loss, and good language and social skills. Over the last five years, however, her illness had progressed because of her strokes, and she now needed help with daily activities, so she had a live-in aide.

"How long has she been vomiting?" I asked. "What color is it?"

"Since this morning," Luke said. "It's bright red."

"Put Polly on," I said.

"Polly," I asked when she picked up the phone, "do you want to go to the hospital?" I knew she abhorred hospitals.

"No," she said.

"You know this is serious. If you stay home, you will bleed to death."

"I know," Polly said. "I'm done."

And I knew it too. Even if we successfully treated this new trauma, I knew that Polly herself would be further diseased, further decimated. The last three years had been a long and painful struggle for us both.

I hurried over to their home. "Steve is

here," Luke whispered in the foyer, nodding toward the bedroom. Steve was Polly's physician. "He wants Polly at the hospital immediately. He wants us to call 911."

"And you, Luke?"

"I'm with Polly. She's been just as brave as can be." Luke's eyes teared up.

"This is a treatable problem," Steve said when I walked in.

"Yes," I said, "but she is going to be worse off afterward."

We went back and forth like this for half an hour. Steve's points were good ones, and I'm sure most of my colleagues would have agreed with him. What I was proposing was not the medical norm. Annie's pleading face in her flapping blue housecoat sprang to my mind. A good medical decision is a good human decision, I reminded myself, and stuck to my course of action. In the end, Steve acquiesced.

Even so, I felt wobbly and unsure. Steve had decades more experience as a physician than I did. What if he was right and I was wrong? What if it was wrong to agree with Polly and let her go, wrong to let her die? I had never helped anyone die before. How would I go about doing it? There were many colleagues I could ask to help me help Polly live, but I couldn't think of anyone to call to help me help Polly die. I could hand her off to a hospice team, of course, an end-of-life, medical cleanup crew. But this felt like a shirking of responsibility, an abandonment of Polly in her time of need, just so I would be spared the discomfort. It felt cowardly to opt out.

I told Luke to alert everyone in the family. The time, I said, had come.

"How long?" Polly asked me.

I didn't know how to answer the question. "It could be a few days," I said. "I will make sure that you stay comfortable."

"Okay," Polly said, squeezing my hand.

A day later, the bleeding stopped, and Polly was drinking only water.

"How are you doing?" I said.

"Cramps, a lot of cramping," Polly said, holding her belly, her face tightening with each abdominal spasm.

"I am going to give you a bit of morphine," I said. "Just a little to help with the cramps." I was nervous, because it was the first time I'd had to prescribe morphine to someone who was dying. I had a lot of experience giving it to patients in pain, but never in a palliative setting such as this, where I was treating the pain alone, not the illness.

By the third day, Polly was barely speaking. Her sons were there with their wives and children, everyone milling around the apartment. The mundane activity felt curiously comfortable and more palatable than the clinical sterility of hospital death scenes. Luke lay next to his wife, propped up with pillows on his side of the bed, exhausted.

By the fourth day, Polly was refusing water and sucking weakly on ice cubes that her aide placed between her parched lips. Her skin was drier, but her heart still thumped steadily in her chest. Her breath was clear, her pulse strong. *Oh God!* I thought. *What if I've been wrong in going along with Polly's wishes? If she was so sturdy of constitution, perhaps I should have insisted on stemming her bleeding.* But it was too late; the die was cast.

Polly awoke briefly and looked around and greeted her children by name.

"How long?" was everyone's question once Polly dozed off, presumably out of earshot. As a side note, this idea of someone not hearing when asleep or unconscious worries me. The muscles of the human ear are the only muscles, aside from those in the eye, that are not paralyzed when we dream. When I am with patients in the ICU, or presumably unconscious patients, I keep in mind that the patient, regardless of their impaired level of alertness, may be hearing and responding emotionally to what I am saying.

In my best approximation of a reassuring, priestly voice, I said, "Not long now."

On Saturday morning, I found to my dismay that Polly was still alive, which meant I had to face her family and continue to pretend that I knew what I was doing. I was filled with guilt that I, her doctor, was not delighted that she was alive. It was not until a few years later that I realized that wanting the dying to be over is not the same as wanting someone to be dead.

I was filled with dread and completely stressed, not to mention sleep deprived. I knew it was unprofessional to be so attached and to cry over a patient. Clinical detachment is valued in medicine. Yet my connection to Polly helped me view things from her perspective, as well as from the perspective of a physician. After all, like all good doctor-patient relationships, ours was a human relationship first. I allowed myself, finally, to break down within the safety of my own home. Then I composed myself and went to see her.

When I finally arrived at her noisy, lively, crowded apartment — so different from the feel of an ICU where she could have been — I saw that Polly's eyes had shrunk into her face. Her lids were closed, and when I lifted them, her corneas had an opaque covering like a spiderweb. Her skin was tight and pulled away from her face, and her lips were dry and peeling. I dabbed some Vaseline on Polly's lips and left soon afterward. What else could I do?

When I got to Polly's apartment the next morning, I found that she had died just a few minutes before. It had been six days from the beginning to the end, our last journey together. Polly's family surrounded her in her bedroom, making plans for the funeral, for trips home, and for the future. The waiting was over, and everyone thanked me. Even Steve, her other physician, hugged me.

I half expected to hear the sound of a champagne cork going off any minute, glasses raised to cheer a life well lived.

ANNIE AND POLLY'S LEGACY

It took me awhile to sort out and recover from the personally draining experience of helping Polly die. I remember seeking counsel from a few older, more experienced colleagues. Fortunately in the decade since Polly's death, a lot has changed in medicine. Palliative and hospice care are on the rise, but counteracting this movement, the practice of postponing death by medical intervention during the terminal months of life is also on the rise.

Since Polly, I have tried to treat my patients' medical illness at home whenever possible. I also do my best to honor the wishes of my patients and their families to die at home. I make sure that I have conversations with families and with patients about their end-of-life wishes well ahead of time. I have been teasingly referred to as the Angel of Death by some of my colleagues because of this, but I take that as a compliment. It feels like a badge of honor in a specialty dealing with chronic illness.

I also make sure that I discuss health care proxies, in which a patient designates one or more people to make health decisions on their behalf should they not be able to do so. I discuss living wills, which lay out a patient's wishes in the event of an illness, including respirators, tube feeding, and other methods of maintaining life. When a patient is gravely ill, I will also discuss medical orders for life-sustaining treatment (MOLST) forms that are signed by the physician, patient, and family members, and give even more specific instructions about medical treatment and resuscitation. All this helps prepare everyone for the death of the patient in as painless a way as possible.

GETTING TREATED WHILE
LOUNGING AT HOME

Marion was 77 when she first came to see me, at her husband's behest, for progressive memory loss that began when she was 74. She wore a tailored suit, her hair was perfectly coiffed, her fingernails were neatly manicured, and draped on one arm was her cute black-and-white Pekingese, Rosie. Rosie was fiercely protective of her owner, and immediately snapped at me when I shook Marion's hand. In subsequent years, she seized every opportunity to try to bite me. Even in her dotage, she would totter toward me with a toothless snarl.

Halfway through my examination, Marion, who was of Eastern European heritage and spoke five languages, waved one arm toward my desk while Rosie perched on her other arm and said airily, "Dahling," she said airily, "do we really need to go through all this? Why don't you tell me what's wrong? Put me on some pills, give me a shot, and I'm done."

I tried to explain to Marion that it wasn't quite as simple as all that. I told her that she would have to go through tests and we would have to figure out what the problem was before I could treat her effectively.

Once more, she simply waved her hand, on which flashed several impressive diamond rings — gifts from her husband, Donnie. He might have been husband number four, but they had been married for twenty years, and he was absolutely besotted with Marion.

"Dahling," Marion purred, "you look very young to me, but I'm sure I can trust you, because Donnie says so. I have no time for this. Take a good look! Do you see anything wrong with me?"

I admitted that she looked marvelously well put together.

"Well then. Am I good to go? Can I tell Donnie that everything is good?"

It went on in this vein for a while. Eventually, after much coaxing, she agreed to get tested. I saw Marion again for a follow-up diagnostic visit and told her that she had slowly progressive Alzheimer's with mild-moderate memory impairment and good language, social, and life skills. She was outraged.

"What do you mean old-timer's disease?" she said, mispronouncing Alzheimer's as some people do. "That's for old people! I'm not old! You don't know anything! I'm going to go home and tell Donnie that I need another doctor."

She marched out with Rosie growling at me over her shoulder, even angrier with me than usual for upsetting her mother.

Marion stayed my patient at the behest of her husband, and as time went on, her condition slowly got worse. She suffered a few strokes, which hastened her decline. By the time she was 84, I had started to visit her at her home because she refused to go out unless it was for a good reason, such as dinner with her husband or the opera. From Marion's point of view, a doctor's office visit did not make the cut.

On my visits to her home, Marion would let me in, then sprawl on a chaise longue in her living room with Rosie perched on one arm, the dog's teeth dangerously close to my stethoscope as I tried to examine Marion.

One morning, I arrived before Donnie left for work. Despite being in his late eighties, Donnie had not yet retired. As he left the room after kissing her good-bye, Marion cried out, "Donnie boy! Donnie boy! Don't go yet!"

With Rosie still on one arm, she leaped out of the chaise, from which she had flat-out refused to move for me a few minutes before, procured a comb, and smoothed his hair into place.

"There," she said, patting his suit jacket. "Now you look even more handsome."

Marion's sparkling personality never faded. Every time I arrived at her home, she'd pat the chair beside her and say, "Oh, it's you again. Enough of this doctor nonsense! How many men have you had recently, dahling?"

I enjoyed my visits with Marion, but by the time she was 88, she was much less talkative. Donnie had died, and Rosie had followed some time thereafter. Marion required round-the-clock care, which her daughter was in charge of coordinating.

Marion needed to walk, but refused to. Her daughter and I conspired to get the hunkiest physical therapist we could find, to motivate her to exercise. This worked for a few years, until even Mr. Hunk couldn't get her to leave her chaise.

By the time Marion was 90, she was mute and unable to walk or sit up, but every day, her caregivers dressed her up, right down to her snazzy heels, and helped her to her chaise. She received excellent care and did not develop a single bedsore despite being bedridden, and suffered just two bouts of pneumonia. Ordinarily, pneumonia is common in cases like Marion's, where patients move little and are fed in bed, increasing the risk of aspirating food particles into their lungs. Between the ages of 85 and 93, when she finally died, Marion had two more strokes and multiple urinary tract infections, and also developed seizures. We were able to treat all this at home, including drawing blood and obtaining urine specimens when needed.

Part of our success in treating Marion at home can be attributed to her daughter, who had agreed that even if Marion was in much distress, she would not call 911. This can be a tricky and painful decision to make for the caregiver, which is why I discuss it with patients and families well ahead of time. In Marion's case, everyone was aware of her dislike of hospitals and doctors, so the decisions were easier to make. In the last two years of her life, there were at least a dozen close calls, times when Marion would stop eating for a day or two, or run high fevers, or when she developed seizures. Throughout, I counseled her daughter and the live-in paid caregivers to stick to our plan, which we did until she died at home in her own bed at age 93.

Marion, like Polly, lived the best life she possibly could under the circumstances, and died a good death, avoiding hospitalization.

Such home-based health care is covered by insurance and available to all of us, although, as I mentioned before, physician home visits are poorly reimbursed. Along with delivering high-quality, in-home care, we also saved society a significant number of health care dollars.

NOT CALLING 911 IS HARD TO DO

It can be difficult to resist the urge to call emergency services when a loved one's health seems to be in danger, as Susan, the daughter of my 94-year-old patient Isabelle, discovered.

Isabelle was a tiny woman, about four feet eight inches, who loved high heels. When she first came to me at 86, I diagnosed her with slowly progressive Alzheimer's disease with moderate memory loss and excellent verbal, social, and life skills.

She was a professional florist, spending her life making beautiful bouquets. She was so talented that she had received letters commending her fantastic flower arrangements from the last eight American presidents. One of the fun things about Isabelle's visits was watching her niftily readjust the flowers on my desk, changing an ordinary bouquet into a masterpiece in just a few seconds — an artist at work.

About three years after her diagnosis, Isabelle required an aide a few hours a day to remind her to take her medications and to help with cleaning and chores. Now 94, she had twenty-four-hour care but still went out socially every week.

One day, she tottered into my office wearing her signature high heels for her usual visit along with her daughter Susan. On this visit, Susan was very concerned about her mother's dental hygiene.

"Her gums started bleeding last week," Susan told me.

When I looked into Isabelle's mouth, I discovered that in fact something more serious was happening.

Upon further questioning, I learned that Isabelle had also been complaining of severe stomach cramps. I sat down beside her and said, "Isabelle, there is nothing wrong with your mouth. It's more serious than that. Your blood pressure is quite low. I think you're bleeding from inside your stomach."

"What does that mean?" Susan asked, quietly.

"It means," I told them both, "that either Isabelle has to go to the hospital to have this taken care of or there is a very real chance of her slowly bleeding to death."

Confronted with this news, Isabelle said,

"I'm ready to die. I don't really want to go to the hospital." The question of hospital versus home was something that Isabelle, Susan, and I had discussed at length in the past, and Isabelle had always advocated for home.

I turned to Susan: "Is that all right with you?"

"Yes," she said.

Normally you wouldn't send someone with internal bleeding home; you would send them directly to the emergency room. This was what Polly's physician, Steve, had argued for many years earlier. But I saw clearly that my role as Isabelle's physician had shifted at this visit. I was no longer charged with keeping her as well as possible. Instead, my goal now was to allow her to be as comfortable as possible as she opted to forgo treatment and, as the result, possibly die at home. Isabelle signed a medical order of life-saving treatment (MOLST) form along with Susan and me. This directive not only specifies what resuscitation efforts one does and doesn't want, but also whether antibiotics and fluids can be used. Isabelle opted out of all such measures. Most patients on the Alzheimer's spectrum are competent enough to make such decisions, and so was Isabelle, despite her poor memory.

As Isabelle and Susan were leaving my office, I realized it might be the last time I would see Isabelle alive. I simply adored this little woman and wanted to say good-bye, but didn't quite know how.

"Isabelle, I'm making an appointment with you for next week, but I want to say good-bye," I said. "In a week, one of us may not be here — it could be me, it may be you. I just want to say good-bye and tell you what a pleasure it has been to take care of you all this time."

It was a hard thing to say, and I found myself choking up.

"Well, it's probably going to be me," Isabelle replied jokingly, ignoring the gravity of her situation, "because I'm a lot older than you are."

"I have really enjoyed getting to know you," I said. "Thanks for all the tips about flower arranging, and thank you for letting me take care of you."

In response to this, Isabelle said something I found deeply touching. "I want you to be around for a long time because I want you to take care of other people like me." We hugged and said our good-byes, and Isabelle left in her lofty heels.

Three days later, on a Saturday afternoon,

a distraught Susan called to say that Isabelle was on the floor, unresponsive. Although Susan had previously agreed not to call 911, she panicked, because Isabelle seemed to be moaning in pain.

"I can't help it," Susan said. "I know we said no hospital, but what if she broke a bone?"

I understood that the reality of seeing her mother in pain was more than Susan could bear. Such panicked departure from previously stated and written directives is not uncommon, even in hospice situations with terminally ill patients. When you see a loved one suffer, it is hard not to do something, even if that something could lead to more suffering.

"Please show the ER doctors the MOLST form," I said, when Susan made it clear that Isabelle was going to the hospital. "Understand that if she does have a broken bone and needs surgery and rehab to repair it, she may not make it. Particularly with her internal bleeding. So even if there are broken bones, Susan, you might want to simply opt to keep her comfortable and free of pain as she and you wanted."

Isabelle went to the hospital, and the doctors there let her go home after reviewing her MOLST form. This form allows ER physicians, who are not familiar with the patient and are charged with saving lives, to allow patients like Isabelle to return home to die. A few hours after returning home, Isabelle died peacefully in her own bed.

Some might think it's a shame Isabelle opted out of life. After all, she was vital and capable until the end. The truth, though, is that she didn't opt out of life. She opted not to be treated for an illness. As a society, we are indoctrinated to leap into action and *do* something. And yet helping Isabelle die by doing nothing was the right thing for Isabelle.

HEALTH CARE PROXIES AND LIVING WILLS

It is rare that patients like Marion, who was immobile the last few years of her life, get to spend their last years at home. More of us — both with and without dementia — will die in nursing homes and hospitals than in our homes. Advance planning helps to prevent disasters and legal issues.

Early in my career, after I graduated from my residency and fellowship, I spent some of my time taking care of patients in a nursing home. This experience left me with a determination to keep my patients out of them whenever possible. The nursing home was also where I met Sam, whose case taught me about the importance of health care proxies.

Sam, 82, was a widower and retired book editor who had specialized in editing historical fiction and made quite a name for himself in the publishing industry during his career. When I met him in the Alzheimer's unit of the nursing home, he was already in a wheelchair because of multiple back injuries.

The unit was filled with caring staff, but many of them were overworked. Wails and screams emanated from different patients' rooms, making for an environment of disquiet and distress. Sam could often be found in the dining room, where there was a television — maybe he was trying to drown out the sounds around him. He was wheeled in for breakfast and often left there for much of the day. He had slowly progressive Alzheimer's with moderate memory loss, good language skills, and moderate impairment of daily living skills. The living skills impairment is what had landed him in the nursing home — he had left the stove on at home one too many times, prompting his family to place him here. When I made my rounds, I would sit and chat with him in that brightly lighted, fluorescent room with no windows.

Sam was confused at times, but at other times, he would have moments of great insight. He once said, "I didn't imagine that it would come to this, that I would be reduced to simply existing. I never thought I would end up in here, but now here is where I am. I want to be home."

He would gaze at me with his eyes, once a deep brown, now clouded over with a grayish film. Somehow, this made him that much more forlorn.

As Sam deteriorated, I heard that court proceedings were in the offing because of disagreements between his two daughters. The daughters — both in their fifties, one a physician and the other a lawyer — cared deeply about their father but had despised each other since they were little girls.

Unfortunately, Sam became a pawn in the battle of wills between them. The lawyer wanted her father alive at all costs, but the physician wanted a DNR — do not resuscitate — order on the chart. Because the two were legally in charge of making his decisions, and because they could not agree, the matter went before a judge, who appointed a lawyer to make health decisions on Sam's behalf. The decisions about how Sam would live and how he would die were ultimately made by a stranger. Sam eventually developed pneumonia, was transferred to the ICU of the local hospital, and died after weeks in a coma.

Sam's case is one reason I urge all of my patients to get a health care proxy and to think it through before designating a person. Sam had not designated a proxy, so both his daughters automatically had the power to make his decisions. On occasion, I have seen a patient not wanting to upset their children and designating two or more of them as their health care proxy, even if they have opposing viewpoints. That creates problems, as it surely would have in Sam's case. Because of his daughters' dramatically different perspectives, Sam should have chosen someone who would make decisions that he would feel comfortable with — either just one of his daughters, or a friend or another family member. One piece of advice about choosing a health care proxy: It is best to choose someone in the general geographical vicinity of the patient, although this is not an absolute requirement.

Sam became a part of the statistics that I mentioned earlier — among the 80 percent who died in an institution and not in his own home as he wished. Families place loved ones in a nursing facility either to ensure their safety, as with Sam, or because the burden of care becomes too much. Arlene was another patient whose daughter moved her into a facility for reasons of safety, again with an adverse outcome that Arlene did not anticipate.

Planning for Illness and Death

Here's a list of the documents needed to help ensure that a patient's wishes are honored in the event of serious illness:

Advanced Directive, also Called a Living Will or a Health Care Power of Attorney
- Legal document specifying what treatments to have in the event of an unknown medical emergency; you can also specify a health care proxy here.
- All adults should have one.

Health Care Proxy/Surrogate, Durable Power of Attorney for Health Care
- Lets you appoint a person or people to make medical decisions in the event you cannot.
- If a proxy isn't appointed, usually the legal next of kin, such as a spouse, child, sibling, or parent, will assume this function.
- Form is available online; requires wit-

nesses, but a lawyer isn't necessary.

- Optional extra page allows you to detail wishes further directing the health care proxy.
- All adults should have one.

Medical Order of Life-Sustaining Treatment (MOLST) Form

- Forms are state-specific and available on-line.
- Intended for sick or terminally ill patients.
- Must be signed by the physician and the patient and/or their health care proxy.
- Contains instructions on resuscitation, level of care, and treatments such as antibiotic use.

Do Not Resuscitate Order

- For terminally ill or very sick patients.
- Tells medical personnel not to perform CPR in the event you stop breathing or your heart stops.

SAFETY VERSUS INDEPENDENCE

Arlene, 82, had slowly progressive Alzheimer's disease with mild memory impairment and good language and social skills. Widowed two years previously, she lived alone in a large house in eastern Long Island, her home for four decades. Arlene still drove to the supermarket, cooked, insisted on shoveling the snow in her driveway, and took daily walks on the beach. Her daughter lived in New York City and worried about her mother being alone, with no one to look in on her every day.

Yet Arlene told me, "I wish my daughter would leave me alone. I enjoy being at home. I have neighbors nearby. It's true that I don't see them much in the winter, but the mailman checks on me, and I don't feel alone or lost. My daughter yells at me because I don't get fresh milk, but I'm not one to throw things out."

Arlene eventually acceded to her daughter's entreaties and moved into a posh assisted-living facility in the city, much to her daughter's relief. But the move worsened Arlene's cognition, making her very confused. She was unhappy with the place, finding something to complain about constantly. Her dementia began to progress more rapidly, and six months later, she tripped outside the door of her new apartment and fell, breaking a hip. Sadly, Arlene did not recover from this fall. She died shortly thereafter in a rehabilitation facility where she was sent after her hip was operated on. Her daughter told me she never learned to walk on her own after the surgery.

In my opinion — and I realize not many people may join me in this — Arlene should have been left in her own home, as she wished. Of course, there was a not insignificant chance that she would have fallen and broken her hip in her own home, but I believe living at home would have offered her a better quality of life until such a time. Moves can accelerate the clinical symptoms of Alzheimer's, not because they accelerate pathology, but because routines are disrupted and it is harder to learn new ones. Think of all the frustrations we go through every time our cell phone operating systems are updated!

How did moving affect Arlene's sense of purpose? Did getting up and shoveling the snow off her front steps and her daily walks on the beach give Arlene more of a sense of purpose than participating in the daily aerobics class at the facility? Arlene was desperately unhappy with the move. How did the unhappiness affect her? We could argue each of these points, but for me the larger question is this: How much do we value safety over independence and quality of life?

As a rule, I advocate for minimizing moves in patients with dementia, because such moves often worsen cognitive symptoms. I have had patients get more disoriented after just visiting with a relative for a weekend, although more often it is longer stays that result in poorer cognition. Disorientation can also occur after admission into a hospital or upon discharge from one, which is one reason I advocate for treatment at home where feasible. Usually, the patient will return to baseline levels of cognition in about two weeks, although in Arlene's case she never returned to the level of functioning she had before her move. Some patients have spent their entire lives summering in Florida or the Hamptons or going up to a weekend home. If that is the case, I would suggest maintaining that routine for as long as possible, keeping in mind that there may be short-term disorientation associated with each move.

THE GOOD GRANDDAUGHTER

Sometimes we have to help a patient die by doing *something* rather than doing *nothing* — by removing life support, for example, or by having the patient discharged from the hospital and allowed to go home. This can be even more difficult than not doing something, because it feels more active than passive, but I found it to be curiously easy when the time came for me to help my grandfather. Although he did not have Alzheimer's, unnecessary medical intervention by a caring yet anxious relative resulted in a tragic cascade of events.

When I was young, my grandfather would ask, "Gayatri, will you take care of me when I am old?"

"Of course, *Thatha,*" I'd reply, with all the fervent conviction of a 7-year-old. To him, I was the perfect grandchild. To me, he was a saint — a powerful man who ran a large company, yet gentle, kind, and deferential, an adult who took me seriously.

I had similarly enriching relationships with my other three grandparents. My headmistress grandmother left me with the short stories of Guy de Maupassant the summer I turned 5, confident I'd figure them out. My other grandfather, tall and soft-spoken, took me on long walks and instilled in me a love of Indian handicrafts. My other grandmother, roly-poly and unschooled, taught me to cook and sew. It is because of them that I chose my subspecialty. I delighted in the treasures an older person could offer. Although I was never able to repay my debt to the three who died when I was young, I did have the chance to do so with my final remaining grandparent.

The years had passed, and both my *thatha* and I grew older, continents apart, he in Chennai, a large city in South India, me in New York. He became 60, then 70, then 80, then 90. Every time I saw him, he strode briskly, usually with a neat little leather folder of his "papers" tucked under his arm. When he retired, he became chief operating officer of my uncle's company.

At 90, he was as healthy as a horse — taking no medications and never having been admitted to a hospital in his life. A lifelong yoga and Ayurvedic practitioner, he was effortlessly fit. Yet on one of my visits, he complained to me that his walk was not quite steady. He felt dizzy when he moved.

"Oh, *Thatha,*" I said, pleased that I knew exactly how to help him. "I can fix it!" I did a bedside procedure on him, repositioning the tiny crystals in his inner ears that had become dislodged, a simple, remarkably effective maneuver.

"Right-o," he said as we said good-bye, once again steady on his feet, cured in minutes with this simple procedure. "I will see you soon!" We were both pleased as punch.

About six months later, I got a call from my uncle's wife. "Your *thatha* is very ill," she said. "He is in intensive care."

"What do you mean?" I asked, dumb-founded.

It turned out that my grandfather had had a recurrent bout of dizziness after being symptom-free for many months, and my uncle had taken him to a neurosurgeon for another opinion. Recurrence is common with this type of positional dizziness, and requires only a repeat of the same simple bedside maneuver I had initially performed. Unfortunately, the neurosurgeon decided to operate to drain some minimal brain fluid that had accumulated with age and that was unrelated to his dizziness. Subsequently, as the result of a complication, my grandfather had bled into his brain.

I took the next plane to Chennai and went directly from the airport to the hospital. When I first saw him, my grandfather was nearly hidden among various bags of fluids and machines, and paralyzed on his left side. He was having seizures and was lucid for only brief intervals. He recognized me right away, although he didn't say anything, smiling wanly instead.

The neurosurgeon arrived and showed me the postoperative MRI. What had once been a healthy brain was now bright with blood on one side. The clot was large, with swelling of the brain, and the future was bleak. I shooed the many relatives out of the room and shut the door, so that my *thatha* and I were left alone.

"It doesn't sound good, and I am not getting any better," he spoke into the silence. "What do you think of my prognosis?"

This was his way — calm, practical, not prone to drama, which is why I so admired him.

"You're right," I said sadly. "The chances aren't good, and even if you eventually get out of here, you'll be paralyzed on one side."

"I've had a good life," he said, "and have lived much longer than your grandmother. It has been nearly twenty years since she left. It's time for me to go and be with her."

"If we remove all these tubes and stop the medication," I said, "you will join her by tomorrow morning."

"Ah, it is that bad, is it?" He grasped the situation quickly. "Okay, let's get on with it."

I have seen end-of-life care in the hospital up close and personal, and it is often one of the saddest, most demeaning chapters of life. The tubes, the constant, painful, and pointless blood draws through paper-thin skin and impossibly skinny veins, the futility of it all as life withers away. I was going to make sure it didn't happen to my beloved *thatha.*

My grandfather and I had a brief meeting with the rest of the family about the plan — everyone was acquiescent, and my grandfather was very much present at the discussion of his death. Upset as I was with my uncle for creating this mess, I noticed how sad he was and how much he adored my grandfather. He had cared for my *thatha* and given him a job that offered meaning and purpose, the great need in the lives of our elders.

At the end, it was my *thatha* and myself, alone in that ICU room. I removed his catheters — the one through his nose into his stomach, the one to his bladder. I removed the irritating cannula that delivered oxygen. I removed the central line to his heart and the intravenous lines in both his arms. He watched me quietly, his hazel eyes intelligent and calm, completely trusting. If I cried, I don't remember it. I remember only a strong sense of purpose, that all my medical education had come to this, helping someone I loved die with dignity. By late Saturday evening, comfortably ensconced in a cheery room with no gadgets beeping and clicking around him, he slipped into a coma. He died peacefully on Sunday morning, and I too was at peace.

I had no qualms about helping my grandfather die, instead going about it with a pervasive feeling of serenity. I believe my relatives agreed to let me do it not only because everyone knew how much I had loved my *thatha* and wanted what was best for him, but also because — thanks to my patients over the years — I was experienced with helping people die with dignity. To me, this is a crucial part of good doctoring and comes with the territory.

Dying at home, which is what most of us wish for, can be achieved through planning — designating a health care proxy, preparing a living will, and signing a MOLST form for those who are more ill. It is essential for the physicians who work with patients on the Alzheimer's spectrum and their families to begin a dialogue about death at an opportune time and leave the door open for further discussions.

Talking about death does not make it any more imminent. Not thinking or talking about death does not postpone or prevent this inevitability. I stress this with families, telling them that I wrote out my own living will at the age of 20 after bearing anguished witness to the trials of the elderly woman I took care of in the ICU as a medical student. In our culture, there is a sanitization of death, a sequestering of it away from life, and this type of compartmentalizing does all of us a great disservice. It behooves us to work through our discomfort, roll up our sleeves, and prepare for the inevitability of death in the best way we can.

CHAPTER 16
GEE, THAT MUST BE DEPRESSING! MY LIFE AS A PHYSICIAN SPECIALIZING IN ALZHEIMER'S — TRIALS, REWARDS, AND LESSONS LEARNED

When I meet people at cocktail parties, dinners, or any social gathering, they often ask, "What do you do?"

"I'm a neurologist," I respond.

"Oh? What kind of problems does a neurologist treat?"

"Anything having to do with the brain, the spinal cord, and the nerves," I reply. "But I specialize in memory disorders, migraines, back pain, and vertigo."

"Memory disorders?" People tend to zero in on this. "You mean like Alzheimer's disease?"

"Yes, and other types of dementias."

"Oh, that must be *so* depressing. How do you manage?"

But I don't find my work depressing at all. Instead, I find it moving, uplifting, energizing. My patients and their families motivate me daily to aspire to be the best physician, neurologist, and person I can. I see my office not only as a strategic war room but also as a haven of sorts, where my patients, their caregivers, and I band together to plot a course that best serves the patient in the long run, functionally and emotionally.

A HISTORY LESSON

One morning recently, I woke up in the doldrums. It was a freezing January day, and I was already off to a late start. I tried to run to the car with my two dogs, but they were having none of it. They refused to hurry along, preferring instead to stop and sniff all manner of aromatic debris strewn on the street. For the next forty-five minutes, we started and stalled our way through three miles of clogged Manhattan traffic, a trip that usually took twenty minutes. When the three of us finally arrived at my office, I was as harried as I could be, with barely enough time to gather myself together before my patients began arriving.

I plopped down at my desk, the dogs at my feet, oblivious and unapologetic in their furry insouciance about their contribution to my state of consternation. Within minutes, it was time for my first patient, Elliot. At 88, he was a retired high-ranking State Department official who had served as an American envoy to many countries over the course of a long and distinguished career. Elliot had slowly progressive Alzheimer's, with moderate to severe memory, language, and life skills impairment, requiring a live-in aide.

I went into the waiting room to greet him: a man of about five feet ten inches, his gray hair brushed back, wearing a tweed jacket over a smart vest, and leaning on a cane. We walked back to my office and sat down. My day, which had been chaotic until that point — what with the traffic, the city trash and noise, the misbehaving dogs — suddenly stilled into a hypnotic hush; it was just Elliot and me, in my silent office, at ten o'clock on a Tuesday morning. He became my sole focus in the moment, as I was his. Our conversation felt almost meditative — everything besides what was happening in that time fell away.

After a frazzle-making morning like mine, yoga would have been nice, but being with my patients was even better.

"So," I said, once we were both comfortably seated across from each other, "what did you think of what's going on in the news?"

Often, this is how I draw patients into a conversation about their memory. I dislike the practice of putting patients through tests during their visits, which immediately puts them on the defensive. I'd much rather test memory conversationally, especially because patients already undergo objective neurocognitive evaluations to establish their cognitive baseline on an annual basis to guide my treatment plan.

"It's bad," Elliot said quietly. "It's bad. . . . In here, it's fine. But out there" — he gestured past my windows — "it's guns, it's war, it's bad."

Then his voice dropped to a whisper, and he said, "When I was little, Hitler was in power, and we had to leave. Hitler was bad. But what's worse now," he continued, "is that some people are as bad as Hitler, but smarter."

Elliot was quiet for a moment before continuing. "I do have faith, though," he said. "If we teach young people well, this could all turn around." He spoke in a quiet, deliberate voice, with the precise diction of someone who had grown up speaking another language.

I thought to myself, *He hasn't given me any specific information about current events, but he conveyed the gist of his thinking.* He related his thoughts about the world in a way that was both inspirational and humbling.

It didn't matter that Elliot's memory and language were poor; he had still given me a personal history lesson. I felt fortunate to be in that quiet space, listening and learning from someone so accomplished. My day suddenly became bright, because I was connecting with a patient who was allowing me into his mind. His Alzheimer's was not relevant in this exchange. I wanted to thank him for it at once, so I did.

"Thank you for this history lesson and sharing your perspective," I told him. "You inspire me with your optimism."

He laughed warmly. Because of his language difficulties, I wasn't sure how much he understood of what I was saying, but as a seasoned diplomat, he heard the tone of my voice and responded to that instead. Despite a lifetime of having people hang on his every word, as his language and memory failed him he was far less a part of conversations. But in the space of my office, he knew I was paying attention and rose to the occasion, taking pleasure in our exchange.

My days are full of such profound moments with other human beings that teach me the beauty of every day and the beauty of individual lives. How could this not be uplifting — a real privilege? Of course, there are also numerous occasions of ineffable sadness as a patient's pathology progresses and they lose cognitive skills. Here too, I try my best to connect and to make sure they feel heard as they talk about their losses and their feelings. In bearing witness to their stories, I know I am of help. I see the courage that it takes them to fight through their difficulties to tell me their stories, and I am inspired.

CALLIE'S COURAGE

Although many of my patients on the Alzheimer's spectrum stay stable with appropriate treatment, Callie did not. Yet she struggled through it valiantly, trying to make sense of a world that was increasingly incomprehensible. I was someone on whom she relied to make it less scary. The more understood she felt, even if it was just by one person, the less alone and isolated she felt.

Callie was a 72-year-old retired executive, fine featured, with forthright, almost translucent eyes through which I believed I could peer into her soul. She came to see me for memory loss, accompanied by her husband, Jim. After we had reviewed the tests she had undergone, I told them my diagnosis: Callie had rapidly progressive Alzheimer's, with mild memory loss, moderate language impairment, and good social skills.

Because she was young — in my practice I consider 72 young, 80 middle age, and 85 and above older — we treated Callie as aggressively as possible. In addition to oral medications, she was given immunoglobulin treatments to help modify her brain's immune response to plaque, and transcranial magnetic stimulation (TMS) to help maintain and improve her brain circuitry.

Callie held her own for the first two years, speaking freely to me about what she was going through.

"I suppose I am experiencing the first real depression of my life. I'm basically an upbeat person, but it has been tough," she said. "I've stopped going out and interacting with people. I've kind of fallen off the face of the earth. I'm still trying to read daily and to understand what I am reading. I get crazy when I can't do something I used to do, and then I don't let it rest until I can."

"Give me an example, Callie," I said.

"The computer is more difficult than it

used to be. I used to be the person saying, 'Are you having a problem? Let me see what I can do for you.' Now *I'm* the person who has the problem. Part of my issue is how nervous I get when something like this happens. I tend to go hide. I have gone days without answering my emails. And that never used to be the case.

"Jim has been a little perturbed by my state and is not letting me do things, like entertaining. We used to do a lot of entertaining. He thinks I'll make mistakes or do something embarrassing. I have to push back at him when he does that, when he tries to protect me by taking over."

"Has that been effective?" I asked.

"Sometimes, for brief periods," Callie said, laughing wryly. "Jim and I have been married for fifty-two years and we don't have time for serious changes in behavior. I am really not a depressed person in my real life, but I don't like what is hanging over me."

"What do you feel is hanging over you?"

"Not knowing who I am and still living." Callie started to tear up. "That is the most hurtful part. I want to have my own dignity."

Three years into her illness, Callie's Alzheimer's had progressed. She lost her ability to write and needed assistance getting dressed. Jim had to do more to help her, and she resented it. She began to have much more trouble communicating with him, although he tried his best to understand her. Callie began to use me as an interpreter and go-between, to help in sharing her feelings and needs with him. In this way, Callie, with some help, created more of a sense of togetherness with her husband and less of a sense of loneliness. Jim also began to use me to help him better understand Callie's behavior, which at times seemed inexplicable to him.

She had a way with words even as her illness progressed and she knew I would listen and try my best to understand what she was feeling. When she came to see me, she would initially fumble, but then in clear and lucid sentences let me know what she was going through.

"I am not a dog on the street!" Callie said angrily once, seemingly out of the blue.

I found out that Jim had taken to leading her gently by the arm whenever they were away from home. "You don't want to be led?" I asked.

"That's exactly right!" Callie exclaimed. "I've proved I can do things on my own. I'm functional. I know I forget sometimes. Jim sees the page, but not the book," she concluded.

I had Jim come back into my office and explained these issues to him, with Callie present.

"Sometimes I get angry," she said, and thumped at her chest. "I get angry with myself first, then with him." She pointed to Jim while still looking at me. "I know that my reasons may not be right, but it feels right, completely real. I feel contained, like I need approval from the chief judge, like I am in prison."

Jim was clearly shocked — he had never seen himself as a judge or a prison guard as he cared for her. But he saw now how Callie felt. Callie, who had always had a strong streak of independence, Ms. Take Charge, was now being told what to do and when and how to do it, and was being evaluated on her abilities on a daily basis by Jim.

Inadvertently, by virtue of being a diligent caregiver, Jim was being viewed as a prison warden. He realized that he would have to let go and let Callie do more on her own, even as he feared for her safety in doing so. He agreed to stop leading her around by the arm, even though he fretted that she would fall.

Once Callie was sure that Jim understood, she let him into her mind a little more. "I didn't think that people with what I have could hurt, but I do," she said, looking at Jim. "How can I feel happy when my life is falling apart? I am an after person. I am here and I am never going back."

Callie began to cry and Jim got out of his chair, lifted her up from hers, and held her, rocking her gently, comforting them both. Callie let herself be held, all the fight out of her, resting her head on his shoulder, finally feeling understood. I knew that Jim now more clearly felt her struggles and would be less likely to take her outbursts of anger personally. By being there and listening to what Callie was experiencing without judgment, I helped her open up and tell her husband what she was going through, which brought them closer together in this, the toughest fight of their lives.

Callie's memory loss was still mild, but her language and living skills difficulties continued to worsen. She could still acerbically comment on the ongoing presidential race, describing the candidates as "operators," and critique operas she had just seen, including the sets and costumes, but she had trouble finding her way to the bathroom. Part of my work with Callie was to point out to her, in as many ways as I could, that despite these many changes, she was still, at her core, Callie: opera lover, weaver of words, perfectionist, beloved by her husband. I found this technique to be reassuring to Callie, as it is with many patients who are terrified of "losing" themselves in the disease.

I am constantly touched by the efforts Callie made to share her experience of her illness with me and by her faith in me. Not a very trusting woman, she put her trust in me. "You will do your best," Callie proclaimed. "Work your magic and make it better."

In the end, although I was not able to keep Callie as stable as either of us would have liked, I was able to get her to a place without anxiety and inner torment. I was able to determine the right doses of the right combination of medications so that she felt safe, even "good."

"I used to be hard to live with," Callie told me when I saw her recently. "Now I am semihard to live with. What I hear above the music is all right."

Callie continues to fight the fight as this book goes to press, speaking more haltingly but still full of spirit and courage. Sometimes she moves me to tears, and at other times she makes me laugh out loud. She has wrestled with her moods and her fears as she has dealt with the journey through Alzheimer's, and I have been in it with her, guiding her the best I can. It is because of men and women like Callie that my job matters to me.

A BEAUTIFUL FACE

As I reflect on my career, many patients like Callie come to mind — patients who have imparted life lessons to me, making me smile or cry or both.

Dia was 82, a small woman with bright green eyes. A retired social worker, she immigrated to New York from Cuba in the 1950s. I saw her for her slowly progressive Alzheimer's with mild memory loss. She would walk into my office with a big smile and say to me in her heavily accented English, "Dr. Devi, old age has an ugly face."

"No, no!" I'd protest. "No, Dia! You are beautiful!"

She would sigh and say once more, "You don't know what you're talking about. You wait until you get old. Old age has an ugly face."

I remember hearing this from her when I was 29, and 30, and then 31 and 32. Eventually Dia died, but after that, whenever I thought of old age, I remembered her voice and her incongruously pretty face, telling me, "Dr. Devi, old age has an ugly face."

The wonderful thing about my practice is that these types of assertions often get flipped upside down by other teachers, by other patients. This particular contention about aging was upended by Helen, a 92-year-old former teacher with slowly progressive Alzheimer's disease. She had dyed black hair that she wore pulled back in a tight, severe chignon. Her black eyebrows had been tattooed in place, arching over her sharp, piercing dark eyes. She hated coming to my office because she didn't believe anything was wrong with her, but her daughter dragged her there every few months for a regular checkup.

I loved seeing Helen. As soon as she got over her initial reluctance at each visit, we had the most fascinating discussions. On one particular occasion, we were talking about her past.

"The wonderful thing about my life is that I've always been adored. Men, women, my students — they all loved me," she said, shaking a beautifully manicured finger in my direction. "Now, that's a quality you really should appreciate, if you have it. I used to look like that actress. What's her name? Elizabeth . . . Elizabeth . . ."

"Elizabeth Taylor?" I offered.

"Yes, that's the one," Helen said, nodding. "From the time I was very young, people would tell me how much I looked like her. I grew up knowing that I was beautiful. It's not something I thought about; it's the way I was. As I grew up, bad things happened to me." She shrugged. "I was married to a dirty, cheating bastard whom I had to divorce. I'm sure I was miserable after the divorce, but I don't remember much of it now. I remember being married to my second husband, who was a good man. It must have been a good marriage, because I don't remember anything bad about it at all."

"What about getting older?" I asked Helen. "When beautiful women get older, they are often concerned about losing their looks."

"What do you mean?" Helen exclaimed, completely taken aback by my question. "Look at me! Don't you think I'm beautiful? What if I'm ninety-two? I'm still beautiful! I've never lost my looks."

I looked at her and I had to agree. Even at almost a century old, Helen was gorgeous, thanks to the sparkle in her eyes and the vivaciousness with which she carried herself.

Suddenly, her voice dropped to a whisper, and she offered up another pearl. "The important thing about life is that you have to stop and savor it when good things happen to you. I always have, and you always should. Most people take the good things that happen in their lives for granted. Never make that mistake. Stop and relish that moment."

Dia and Helen taught me the importance of narrative, not only in how we view the world, but also in how we view ourselves. Dia, despite her ebullience and her beauty, thought herself old and ugly, whereas Helen had a dramatically different perspective. The stories we tell ourselves and those we tell others shape who we are. I know stories can be changed — that's the storyteller's prerogative. What will be my story? That, my patients have taught me, is entirely up to me.

BURNING OUT

Despite the uplifting daily encounters with patients like Callie and Helen, sometimes even paid caregivers like myself can experience burnout, given the intensity of what we witness on a daily basis. I first noticed it one afternoon as I was listening to Jerry's story, many years after I had started practicing in my specialty.

"He started to see little people every-where," Jerry's wife, Jackie, was saying as he watched her. "He thought there were people on the lawn, climbing up through the windows, crawling out of the radiators. He was calling the police every other minute. I was in the kitchen preparing dinner once when the cops arrived, and I had no idea why they were there. Isn't that so, Jerry?" she said, looking over at her husband.

Jerry, 82, was a retired schoolteacher, tall and slender, impeccably dressed, freshly shaven, his gray hair combed back. Jackie, also 82, was also elegantly attired with a fine hat. I admired the care with which people of that generation dressed, even for a doctor's visit.

Jerry looked over at his wife. "Yes, honey," he said. "Now I know it wasn't real, but at the time, it seemed real to me."

"Yesterday," Jackie said, "he thought he saw a little dog in our living room. We're not even dog people!"

Watching them, I realized their relation-ship was going to change over the next few years as Jerry developed more symptoms of Lewy body dementia. Patients with this type of dementia can experience vivid visual hal-lucinations, and often have good insight into the experience once the actual episode is over. The good news is that these symptoms can be effectively treated with medications.

I had already silently made my preliminary diagnosis, having listened to similar stories over the years, although it would need to be confirmed by a thorough evaluation and testing. But the excitement of formulating a possible diagnosis in Jerry, of figuring out how to treat the various nuances — not just of the disease, but of the specific way this illness affected this particular person — had vanished in the previous year.

I didn't enjoy going into the office anymore. I felt like a machine, seeing one patient after another. Their questions and complaints merged into one. I no longer felt the connection that I treasured between myself and my patients. This was reflected in my interactions with them, which had become less personal. I believe my patients sensed the change — they no longer asked me, "How's it going, Doc?" or "How's the dog?" or "Oh, you got a new haircut?"

In truth, I had it better than the majority of my colleagues. I designed my office to be homey, eschewing medical furniture for couches and comfortable chairs, serving cookies and fresh coffee with milk. I brought my dogs to work with me. I hired like-minded staff, who truly cared about our patients and their families. I was not bound by many of the constraints of insurance companies, and I could describe myself as successful in my practice. I was making a living, doing what I loved to do, and I had nothing to complain about.

Yet there I was, feeling more and more unfulfilled and unhappy. I discussed this with my family, colleagues, and close friends, all of whom advised me against making any rash decisions, yet still the idea of a big move, perhaps into something totally different, like farming, became more and more attractive.

Burnout among physicians is high, with doctors leading a list of eleven professions in suicide rates. In one large study, burnout symptoms were present in more than half of the more than seven thousand American physicians surveyed, and a third of them felt cynical with patients, sometimes treating them as objects. How ironic, as most of us had chosen medicine because we cared about people and wanted to help them. At this point in my career, I recognized immediately, and with horror, that I fit the profile of the burned-out physician.

It took me almost a year of self-examination to find the root cause of my unhappiness. It came to me suddenly, out of the clear blue. I realized that I was missing the most important ingredient that I had enjoyed in my practice — the time to chat and connect with my patients.

When I finally figured it out, I was taken aback by the simplicity of it. Over the years my practice had become so busy that I had almost no downtime to spend with my patients. I had little opportunity to get to know them as people. I realized that personal interaction with my patients fueled my joy in my practice.

I wanted time to shoot the breeze with my patients about things that had nothing to do with medicine, nothing to do with illness, nothing to do with treatment, so that I could know them and relate to them as people, rather than as just patients. And if they chose, they could know me and relate to me as a person rather than as just their physician.

The way that I resolved this problem was simple but effective. I added a five-minute cushion to the end of each regular patient visit. I call that extra window my "chitchat time." Patients are not aware that it's there and we may not use it, but it allows me to take time to feel more connected with them if I feel we need it. In those few minutes, we can talk about anything — pets, hobbies, clothes, family, whatever comes up.

PERSONAL CONNECTIONS

Ultimately, I feel a lot more useful when I maintain personal relationships with my patients, because I feel more attuned to them as whole people. It makes for a richer experience for both me and my patients and ultimately, in chronic illnesses, leads to better care. To be a part of someone's life during stressful and fraught periods requires a measure of connection that I could not give in a solely clinical environment. Detachment may work for some doctors, but it doesn't work for me. I allow myself to cry when a patient dies, and I cry when I cannot help them. But the sense of reward and happiness I feel when something I do helps a patient is enormous.

Along those lines, I am a strong believer in the importance of touch and the healing power of the human hand. Many of my older patients go untouched by others, which is deeply sad. Some are touched but only through gloves, handled like an object. I try my best to have my patients feel as physically close as possible in a medical setting. It helps that I'm a very physical person. I like to hug my patients, a different type of contact from a task-oriented one like taking a blood pressure reading. I like to sit next to them, whether we are in the examining room or the waiting room. This type of human physical contact — within a medical setting — also helped to alleviate my burnout.

My own caregiver burnout taught me valuable lessons that I can now impart to the caregivers of my patients. Burnout is insidious and can creep up on you, becoming a pervasive feeling that you can't quite put a finger on. I had always had a deep respect and admiration for many of the caregivers I encountered, but after my own experience of burnout, this feeling deepened. I, after all, was not wedded to the job, but many of them literally were; I could go home at the end of the day or go away on vacation, but many of my caregivers had no way out. I try my best to instill in caregivers the importance of keeping their relationship with the patient alive while still doing their "job." This is crucial in avoiding burnout.

These days, I find it increasingly difficult to figure out when I am doing my best as a physician. There are always new drugs to try, new technologies to use, and endless possibilities for treatment modalities. Now more than ever, when we have so much science at our disposal, medicine remains an art. The array of options makes medical decision-making ever more nuanced. How do we decide on the best recipe for the healthiest possible life for each individual patient with their own particular version of Alzheimer's? A patient's definition of health may be different from mine. For one patient, continuing to go to dinner parties may be the definition of health, for another it may be driving, and for another it may be being left alone to do as they damn well please in their own home, thank you very much. Letting my patients know that their wishes are no less important, even if idiosyncratic, has become one of the pillars of my approach to dementia care.

SAYING THANK YOU

My days are full of stories, human in their glorious ups and their messy downs. By allowing me into their lives, my patients and their caregivers have sculpted me into a better physician and, I hope, a better mother, partner, friend, and human being. When I was nearing the tenth anniversary of starting my own private practice, my thoughts turned nostalgic. I felt immensely grateful and wanted to share how I felt and thank the people who had made it happen — my patients and their families. So I mailed a thank-you note to my patients.

PRACTICE REFLECTIONS

"It's more important to know what person the disease has than what disease the person has."
— HIPPOKRATES OF KOS

May 17, 2009, marks my tenth year in solo practice, and my thoughts turn inward. My great-grandfather sent out his practice announcement to the "citizens" of Tanjore, an ancient city-state in South India, more than a hundred years ago. So much has changed in the practice of medicine since then. But the joy of caring for patients is the same.

I have been a part of many families as they transitioned through difficult times in their lives, and have cared for parents and children, for siblings and spouses. Work brings me a daily sense of deep and abiding gratitude. The grace of my patients and their families has been a revelation. In truth, I have been blessed in having some of the most wonderful patients in the world. They have taught me all manner of things, great and small. I have amazing mentors and stellar colleagues, who are never too busy to give me advice or lend me a hand, an ear, or sometimes even a shoulder. My own family has been unbelievably magnificent.

I am not sure what the future will bring, but I am overjoyed to mark the passage of ten of the most fulfilling years of my career. I wished to celebrate it in some small way with the folks who made it happen, hence this letter. A journey started with trepidation a decade ago has become a most meaningful, humbling, and wondrous thing. In a way, my practice feels much like my great-grandfather's must have, more than a hundred years ago: a small city-state of patients and their families, physicians and colleagues, students and teachers, a community I am privileged to be a part of. The voyage continues, but this is my opportunity to say a most heartfelt thank-you!

About two years after I had sent out my note, I was talking to Maggie, a patient with rapidly progressive Alzheimer's disease. We were trying to figure out what new prescription her internist had written for her. She was carrying an overstuffed handbag, which is not uncommon in dementia, as patients worry about what they might forget and place all sorts of "important" things in it. She had lost her prescription inside it, and so she emptied her capacious bag. Out came two wallets — again not uncommon in patients with dementia — Maggie's keys, many rubber-banded wads of bills that needed paying, her checkbook, photos of her grandchildren, and . . . my letter, in the envelope I had mailed it in. I picked it up in astonishment from the pile of items on my desk.

"I loved it," Maggie told me simply, after she figured out what it was.

I realized how much Maggie appreciated that I had shared my feelings about my practice and revealed how much I valued my patients. Many patients on the Alzheimer's spectrum worry that they are a burden — that they are boring, that they may have told that story before, that, in short, they are not wanted, they are not contributing. It gave me great joy to let my patients see that they did matter — to me, to their loved ones, and to their communities; that even as they may pose some difficulties in various ways because of their illness, they still bring knowledge and happiness into the world.

Irene has been dead for eight years now, but whenever she comes to mind, a smile slides across my face. With her infectious laugh and ready wit, she taught me a lot about having the right attitude toward aging. I often wanted to bottle her spirit and dole it out to those in the doldrums.

Shortly before her 95th birthday, seven years into her slowly progressive Alzheimer's, she was in my office, opining in her inimitable way. She was in particularly rare form that day, so I asked her if I could interview her. This tickled her pink. What follows is a verbatim excerpt of our conversation, starting with her description of herself.

"I am a very happy person. I like to laugh, I like to sing, I like to dance. I don't sit and bite my nails and make a tragedy of everything. I can be a comedian at times. I like people. I say hello to everyone, even to strangers on the street." Irene chuckled, then started to sing full throttle from the Broadway musical *Annie.* "The sun will come out tomorrow, tooomorrow. Come what may, tomorrow, the sun will come out tomorrow!"

Irene looked at me with her twinkling black eyes and said, "The sun is still going to come out, if not tomorrow, so a day later. When you go home, you're going to say, 'That's some patient I have.' How many people come in here and sing? That's me. I am not a nag and I don't complain. I am just myself — my disposition, my laughter."

"So that's how you deal with setbacks or problems? Not complaining?" I asked.

"Everybody has bad things happen to them. I lost my husband. I had known him since I was sixteen; it was like I lost my right arm. It's been ten years, but you don't ever get over it. Even now, when I come into the kitchen every morning, there's a big picture of him and I say, 'Hi, sweetheart! I miss you. Did you miss me?' Like I am carrying on a conversation with him.

"All of us know that sooner or later we'll have to go. We're not going to live forever, we're just not. So get over it. Here's something funny about that. I had a neighbor on my floor that died, and I went over when they were sorting through her papers and whatnot. I asked, 'How old was she?' And they said, 'A hundred,' and I said, 'Oh really! Well, I am never moving off *this* floor!' I'm still here, aren't I? Come to think of it, I have a birthday coming up next week, I think."

"How old will you be?" I asked.

"I don't know. I never bother with that sort of thing. If you never saw me before, how old do you think I'd be? And you'd better answer that one correctly!"

"Any more advice?" I asked, evading her question, knowing she was parrying cleverly because she did not remember how old she was.

"Well, marriage is a big one. Everyone carries on about it. I had an excellent marriage for sixty-five years, and it was this simple: Don't be a complainer, be kind, and don't be jealous.

"We enjoyed each other's company," Irene went on. "When he was in business, he used to say, 'Why don't you come to the office?' and he would take me out to lunch. Why should people worry? You're born and then you're gone."

"Who's your favorite person?"

"Myself!" She laughed heartily.

Later, at the end of her visit, I had to give her an injection. Irene said, "You're lucky I took a shower!" Rubbing the sore spot, she added, "You are mean, you know that? But deliciously mean. You must've shot my ass full of liquor. No wonder I'm so funny."

Irene was the classic Alzheimer's cocktail personality conversationalist. She didn't remember her age, but she sure wasn't going to let that impede the flow of conversation. She turned the tables on me instead. Although Irene has been gone nearly eight years, what she taught me will stay with me until I too am gone. She taught me about living, really *living,* rather than just existing, even in the face of adversity and loneliness. She taught me about the resilience of the human spirit.

SELINA'S FEEDBACK

As we near the end of the book, I thought it would be fitting to share some feedback from a patient on her experience with my practice. I chose Selina because she is a retired nurse who ran a dementia clinic for nearly two decades, so I thought her perspective would be particularly valuable. I had diagnosed Selina, now 70, with slowly progressive Alzheimer's disease two years previously. She had excellent language and life skills with mild memory loss, for which she was being treated with weekly TMS and brain exercises, as well as oral medications. She reflected on the time she had been under my care, contrasting it with her past experience working with patients on the Alzheimer's spectrum. "It was pretty bleak back then," she said. "There was a lot of denial in the medical field as well as in the community. We didn't see people until they were eight or ten years into the disease. I loved my work, though. I liked dispensing the knowledge I had, dispelling myths."

"What was the prevailing myth?" I asked.

"The myth was *senility,* that as you get older you get *this.*" She gestured at herself. "That was the number one myth."

A few years after retiring, Selina began to develop the telltale symptoms she knew so well.

"I just knew that something was off," she said. "I would lie in bed and think, *I have Alzheimer's.* I remember my staff and I used to sit in my office and say, give us cancer, give us a stroke, give us anything but dementia. I didn't want to lose myself, which is what I feared most. I didn't want to become a burden. I have never been a very competitive person, but I am competitive about my intellect, and I was terrified of losing it.

"The luckiest day I have ever had was coming here," she continued. "I certainly think I am better now than I was when I started coming to you. The treatments are clearly working, and most days I feel completely fine. But I also appreciate how I feel when I am here at this office. It's easy to sit here and be a part of this experience, which was once so frightening to me. Your staff likes the patients, and it's important to like the patients. No matter how demented people are, they still feel. People feel, and you need to be able to speak to that, and you do a good job with that.

"You see your patients' limitations as their strength," she continued. "When I'm sitting across from you, I know you are not looking at me through the lens of illness. It is not an exchange of 'This is what is wrong with you.' You empower the person to move through the illness and somehow harness it, if possible."

This type of feedback is what keeps me going and motivates me to do what I do. It's why I love my job and cannot imagine doing anything else. It's the type of feedback that allows me to aspire to be a better physician and a better person every day.

As We Part ...

I hope you have enjoyed reading this book and meeting my fantastic patients and their amazing caregivers. I hope I have convinced you that Alzheimer's is a spectrum disorder that exhibits itself and progresses differently in different people, and that it can respond to treatment. I hope you are inspired to reach out and learn from those in your community who may have the illness. I hope that those of you who are reading this book because of concerns for yourself will become proactive and get yourselves evaluated and treated for whatever cognitive issues you are facing.

In the twenty-three years that I've specialized in the field of dementia — five years in full-time academia and eighteen years in my own practice — it's been a rare day that I've come home from treating patients and not felt in some way uplifted. It is also rare for me to feel like I've not been useful. When I come home irritated or upset, it's usually over things that have nothing to do with my patients — bureaucracy, meetings, journal articles that I need to finish writing.

Every day brings gifts in the form of stories, insights, and, best of all, patients who are doing well. I can't think of any other field where I would be as involved in one-on-one, pure human contact as the field I'm in — nor one where such contact is as needed — and for that I'm indebted. It has been important for me to help and encourage patients to see all that they have to offer and all that makes them useful members of society, even if they happen to have Alzheimer's disease.

I believe I have helped patients live fuller

lives and see how much they offer their families, friends, and the world despite — and perhaps even because of — their diagnosis. I let them know how much they have taught me. I have also helped caregivers realize that when they take better care of themselves, they will be better able to take care of their loved ones. In the process, I have learned to take better care of myself. I have seen grace and love in all its shades of beauty.

My work is truly fulfilling and at times nothing short of exhilarating. I'm there to celebrate with my patients when they get better and stay better. I'm there to rejoice with them when they are holding their own. I've officiated at a patient's wedding. I've had one child and one grandchild of a patient named after me.

At other times, my work makes me sad. I am there when patients aren't doing well and when they get acutely ill. Sometimes there's nothing I can do to help them get better or even stay stable. Even in times like those, I try to be of use, because there is one thing that I can still do and that I try to do well: help my patients live with as much joy, purpose, and dignity as possible, regardless of where they fall on the Alzheimer's spectrum.

INDEX

A

Abilify (aripiprazole), 266
acetylcholine, 80, 236
advanced directives, 510
aerobic exercise, 106
agnosia, 295–97
agoraphobia, 259
alcohol, 105–6, 185–87
alprazolam (Xanax), 256–57, 267
Alzheimer's. *See also* diagnosis; memory
    causes of, 41–42
    early symptoms of, 26–27
    early-onset, 199–208, 210
    factors affecting, 17–18
    late-onset, 209–10
    as multifactorial disease, 17–18, 208–10
    preclinical, 49–50, 61–62, 208–10
    prevention of, 107–9, 215–21
    as spectrum disorder, 15, 16–17, 24–28,
        49–50, 61–63
    spectrum-based approach to, 45–49

moves, minimizing, 513–14
multifactorial disease, 17

N

Namenda (memantine), 78, 80–81
Namzaric, 81
National Institute of Aging, 49
National Institute of Neurological Diseases
    and Stroke, 55
neuronal connections, 43
neuroplasticity, 95, 99–100
New York State Committee on Physician
    Health, 155, 174–75
nursing homes
    end of life care and, 506–7
    fear of, 373–76
    ideal, 376–80
    intergenerational, 376–78

O

occupational driving rehabilitation
    specialists, 184–87
off-label interventions, 30–31
olanzapine (Zyprexa), 262, 266, 305
over-learned memory, 151, 168, 170–71

P

pain, 97
paranoia, 300–11, 318
Parker, Dr., 242–45

swallowing difficulties, 294–95
symptoms, 20
synaptic connections, 43–44

T
tangles, 56, 68–69
thank you, saying, 544–47
touch, 474, 542
tracking devices, electronic, 194
transcranial magnetic stimulation (TMS)
    treatments, 78, 81, 93–97, 98–99
trazodone, 267, 281
treatment
  current view of, 38–41
  overview of, 79–82
  positive responses to, 30–33
  reluctance to pursue, 74–77

U
under-diagnosis, 24–25
urinary tract infections, 415, 416–19

V
valerian root, 267, 281
Valium (diazepam), 237, 257, 262, 264,
    267, 280
valproic acid (Depakote), 266
violence, 318, 319–21
vitamin supplements, 81

ABOUT THE AUTHOR

Gayatri Devi, MD, FACP, FAAN is the Director of the New York Memory and Healthy Aging Services and an Attending Physician at Lenox Hill Hospital. She is a board certified neurologist, with additional board certifications in Pain Medicine, Psychiatry, and Behavioral Neurology, and she served on the faculty of New York University's School of Medicine as Clinical Associate Professor of Neurology and Psychiatry until 2015. She is the author of over 50 publications in peer-reviewed journals on the topic of memory loss, as well as the books *Estrogen, Memory and Menopause* (Alphasigma Press, 2000), *What Your Doctor May Not Tell You About Alzheimer's Disease* (Time Warner Books, 2004), and *A Calm Brain* (Dutton, 2012). She lives in New York City.